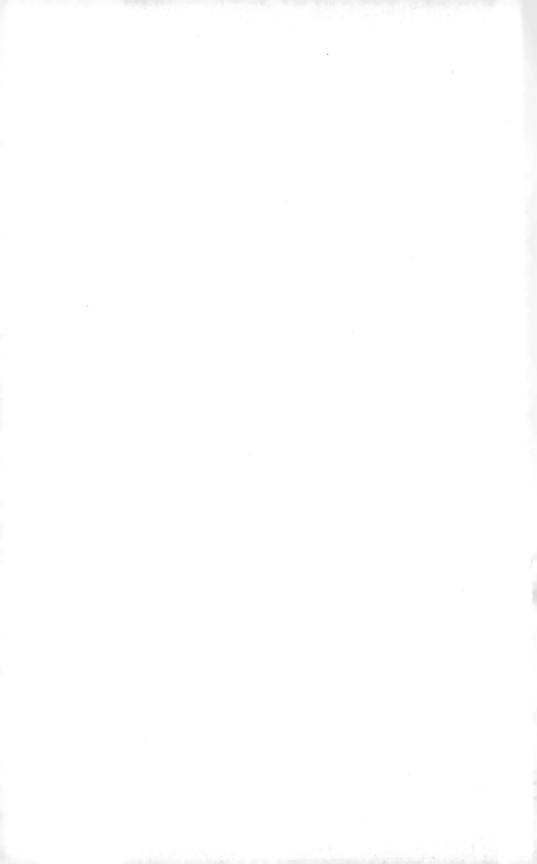

YOUR BEST BODY AT 40+

The 4-WEEK PLAN to Get Back in Shape—and Stay Fit Forever!

By *New York Times* best-selling author JEFF CSATARI and the Editors of **Men's Health**®

LIVE YOUR WHOLE LIFE™

We Inspire And Enable People To Improve Their Lives And The World Around Them

+

This book is dedicated to men
everywhere who realize that,
at 40+, the best years are
yet to come—and that we can
be stronger, smarter, better
than men half our age.

contents

+ACKNOWLEDGMENTS

Writing **Your Best Body at 40+** was very rewarding and motivating, because all those long hours at the computer taught me just how important stretching is to the proper function of a 47-year-old body. And it was a lot of fun, too, as it gave me to opportunity to work with some really smart people. I'd like to say "thank you" to those folks in this space.

First, before a writer can start tapping away on a keyboard, someone needs to say, "Okay, there's a need for this book and we believe in it." Those people are the members of the Rodale family, president and CEO Steve Murphy, and executive vice president of customer marketing Gregg Michaelson—the gatekeepers who ensure that a new project meshes with our company's mission "to inspire and enable people to improve their lives and the world around them." Thank you for believing that this book can help men embrace this most crucial decade proactively by making healthier lifestyle choices. Thanks also to senior vice president and *Men's Health* brand leader David Zinczenko, who cleared the decks and secured the resources to make this book a priority.

Once a book is green-lighted, the actual information gathering begins. I am grateful to the many doctors, researchers, nutritionists, psychologists, and exercise physiologists who graciously shared their time and wisdom through interviews, e-mails, and last-minute phone calls—especially Joe Maroon, MD; Vonda Wright, MD; Mark Moyad, MD; James Kenney PhD; Jeff Volek, PhD; Robert Sapolsky, PhD; Leslie Bonci, RD; Harold Millman, DPT; and Ron DeAngelo. And I am fortunate to have been able to draw on the previous work of the best health and fitness research-ers, reporters, and writers in the world at *Men's Health*, including Peter Moore, Bill Phillips, Matt Marion, Adam Campbell, Bill Stieg, Matt Bean, Matt Goulding, and Eric Adams; and at *Best Life* magazine, Jack Otter, Ben Court, Trevor Thieme, Joel Weber, and Heather Hurlock.

Special thanks to vice president of *Men's Health* books Stephen Perrine and to Bob Love, *Best Life's* former executive editor, who lent considerable editorial direction and helped polish the manuscript. The cover and interior pages were crafted by a talented art director Davia Smith with Emily Reid Kehe, under the direction of *Men's Health* books design director George Karabotsos. Thanks also to the team responsible for the clarity and accuracy of the instructional workout photographs in this volume: photo editor Mark Haddad; photographer Beth Bischoff; exercise consultant Dan Owens; and model and personal trainer Tim Adams, who at 41 can crank out handstand pushups without breaking much of a sweat. Finally, a big thanks to those wizards of production Lois Hazel, Chris Krogermeier, and Debbie McHugh, who delivered this book to press on time. You folks did the heavy lifting.

Jeff Csatari
June 2009

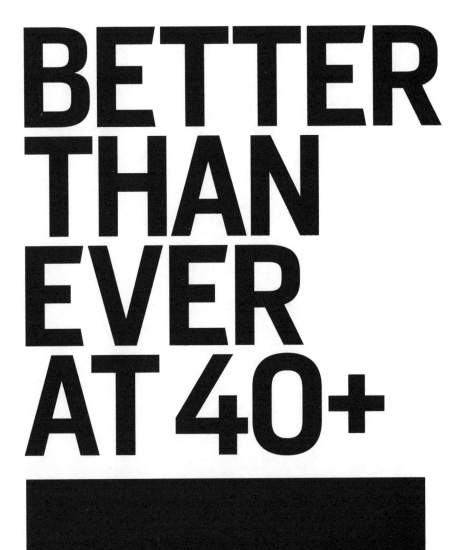

BETTER THAN EVER AT 40+

The 6-Week Plan That Will Help You Get Back Into Shape for Life

 ELCOME TO THE MOST CRUCIAL DECADE OF YOUR LIFE.
Maybe you've just pulled off at exit 40, heading onto the next stretch of your big journey. Or perhaps you're looking at that milestone in the rear-view mirror from a distance of a year or two. Either way, congratulations! You've survived the bad haircuts and boy bands, the blind dates from hell and the slow climb out of the cubicles. You've seen booms and busts—a few of each by now— and you've had your heart broken and healed in any number of ways. Oh, and all that hype about 40 being the new 30? Well, it's actually true—if you play the next 10 years really smart.

For men and women alike, the 40s bring the first great opportunity to reassess, take charge, repair neglect, and remake the rest of your life. Thanks to breakthroughs in medicine, health, exercise, and nutrition, a fortysomething today has a chance to live longer, stronger, and leaner—to remake his body into a sleeker, fitter, stronger version of its younger self. ➡

The other bit of good news is this: You're smarter than you used to be. With the experience, discipline, and savvy you've already acquired, you now possess many of the tools needed to take control of your health and well-being. And you're still young enough to take advantage of them to bend the future to your advantage. If you seize this moment and follow the fitness plan in this book, the next 10—or even 20!—years will be the healthiest, most productive and satisfying years of your life. All you need is a simple strategy to get you back into shape. Lucky for you, that's exactly what this book is about.

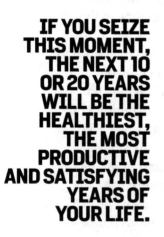

IF YOU SEIZE THIS MOMENT, THE NEXT 10 OR 20 YEARS WILL BE THE HEALTHIEST, THE MOST PRODUCTIVE AND SATISFYING YEARS OF YOUR LIFE.

But first, a reality check. Anyone who's faced down 40 candles on a birthday cake can tell you firsthand that *change happens*. By the time we are in full possession of a fortysomething physique, most of us have lost a few steps, gained a few inches around the middle, and found that we have to work a little harder to keep up with the kids. Even if the bathroom mirror compliments you and tells you that you've staved off many of time's effects on yourself, the proof of time's passage comes in the rounded faces, saggy eyes and jiggling bellies of your friends and co-workers. Is everyone but you getting older? And what about those high school classmates who've tracked you down on Facebook—the ones with the gray hair and the triple chins? Can they possibly be the same age as you? Are we all destined to age that badly?

The answer is no. There is an emerging consensus that everything we thought we knew about aging is false. "The problems typically attributed to aging have less to do with actual aging than with the sedentary way more than 70 percent of people in this country choose to spend their lives," says Vonda Wright, MD, assistant professor of orthopedic surgery at UPMC Center for Sports Medicine, who runs a program called START for people over 40 who want to get back in shape. "It's never too late to build muscle. It's just different. When we were 20, our bodies could do anything to shape up. From 40 onward, we have to be a lot smarter about it. But there's no reason you can't be fitter than you were 5, even 10 years ago."

Your Best Body At 40+

Exercise physiologists, nutritionists, and gerontologists now agree that during the decade of your 40s, men still have enormous potential for getting leaner and stronger, improving energy level and brain function, and transforming decades of bad habits into a healthier lifestyle that will prime them for smooth sailing the rest of their lives.

Think it's too late? Think again. You must have seen some of these men and women at the beach or the gym—the silver-haired surfers and svelte, sexy cougars who look a decade or two younger than their years. And we've all seen what 40+ looks like in professional sports, from baseball to ice hockey and ultimate fighting. In the summer of 2008, American swimmer Dara Torres, at age 41, left the Beijing Olympics with three silver medals. Earlier that year, 46-year-old Chris Chelios helped his Detroit Red Wings take the Stanley Cup. Another 46-year-old, Jamie Moyer, won 16 games as a pitcher for the Philadelphia Phillies, helping the Phils to win their first championship in 26 years.

Still not convinced? Look at Tom Cruise at 46, or Will Smith or Brad Pitt, 44, or Daniel Craig, 41! Consider Laird Hamilton, 45, the chiseled surfing legend, who can beat kids half his age in a beach sprint. Or adventure racer Dean Karnazes, arguably the world's fittest man at 47 years old, who has completed 50 back-to-back marathons!

Well, you're thinking, these folks are freaks of nature, or rich actors who can afford constant body maintenance, right? Wrong again. There are growing numbers of everyday Americans who are incredibly fit at 40+. At least 50,000 of them belong to the 40-and-above rankings of masters swimmers. According to the U.S. Track and Field Association, the number of marathon runners over 40 has increased more than five-fold to more than 162,000. Triathlons have become the sport of choice of the fit 40+ crowd. "People in their 40s make up the fastest growing segment of the sport," says Tim Yount, senior vice president of marketing and communications at USA Triathlon.

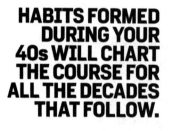

HABITS FORMED DURING YOUR 40s WILL CHART THE COURSE FOR ALL THE DECADES THAT FOLLOW.

But in a man's 40s, health, fitness and sex appeal aren't automatic. Testosterone and growth hormone begin to abate, and metabolism slows. The game gets a little more complicated—and you need to use your wits and wisdom to stay on top of it. But if you make smart tweaks to your fitness and diet plan, and control stress in your work and family life, you'll be set up for the next many years of looking and feeling great.

And that's what makes this your most crucial decade. Whether you spend the next 10 or 20 years looking and feeling your best, or take the slow downhill ride, is now your choice. You don't have a long time to decide. So make your play: Stay with those who believe that aging and physical decline are inseparable and hobble off to middle age, or buck that foolish notion and embrace youth, health, and sexual vitality.

In these pages, we've burned through and boiled down a whole world of scientific research, focusing on the newest information targeted precisely at the 40+ man. And we've created an exercise and eating plan that will change the way you look, feel, and live, today and in the years to come. Plus, we've assembled a dream team of expert advisors who will teach you how to control stress, look your best, and take control by following the advice in this book. In these pages we've gathered all the latest scientific information in a simple, easy-to-follow plan that is guaranteed to turn back the clock and get you in the shape of your life.

The Ultimate 6-Week Plan

You may not be able to recoup your lost 401K losses any time soon, but you can seize control of the things you can improve—your body and your health. And you can do it in as little as 6 weeks, with a smart eating plan and the perfect workout for your body—both of which you'll find in these pages. "The single thing that comes close to a magic bullet, in terms of its strong and universal [health] benefits, is exercise," says Frank Hu, MD, professor of nutrition and epidemiology at the Harvard School of Public Health.

Don't worry if you're new to the game. Once you experience the uplift that exercise and eating right bring to your body, your mind, and your self-confidence, you'll find plenty of motivation to keep it up for the rest of your life. The 10 chapters in this book, which cover all aspects of the fit-at-40+ lifestyle, were written to help you do just that.

Conquering the Crucial Decade

The time to get back in shape is now. The 10-year span between the ages 40 and 50 is critically important because the habits formed during this decade will chart the course for all those that follow. In your twenties and thirties, you had the luxury of time. You could eat badly, stay out late, work out when the spirit moved you. You could let yourself go without worrying much about your health. Frankly, that's no longer the case. At the very least, living like that will pile on the pounds. More likely, your health will suffer. Heart disease and diabetes can hunt you down if you're not vigilant. Consider the statistics: More than a quarter of Americans over age 30 are insulin-resistant, a condition known as "metabolic syndrome," or "pre-diabetes," and on the verge of full-blown diabetes. That figure rises to 40 percent of the American population over the age of 60. And once you have diabetes, odds are that you will have it the rest of your life. Some people can reverse it with much effort and commitment, but most can only hope to manage it with diet and medication. And managing it is difficult, too. Seventy-five percent of people with diabetes will die of cardiovascular disease.

But you can avoid that fate with very little effort. In a landmark fitness survey known as the Nurses' Health Study, researchers found that moderately intense exercise—that means walking for a half hour to an hour each day—lowered the risk of developing type 2 diabetes by up to 40 percent. Just walking! Dr. Hu, the Harvard researcher and epidemiologist involved in that study, says nothing is quicker or more effective for preventing diabetes than exercise.

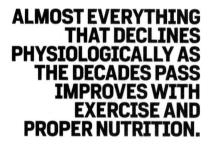

ALMOST EVERYTHING THAT DECLINES PHYSIOLOGICALLY AS THE DECADES PASS IMPROVES WITH EXERCISE AND PROPER NUTRITION.

Exercise not only builds muscle but it impacts nearly every organ in the body. It builds new capillaries in the skeletal muscles, heart, and brain. Red blood cells increase in number, improving oxygen transport. Blood pressure and resting heart rate go down, reducing the stress on the heart and arteries. The left ventricle of the heart increases in size and becomes more efficient at pumping blood.

The best news of all? Almost everything that declines physiologically as the decades pass improves with exercise and proper nutrition. What does that mean for you? It means you have the opportunity to change your life right now. Every journey begins with a single step, which you have already taken. Congratulations. Your new life begins on the next page.

+JUST LOOK AT WHAT YOU HAVE TO GAIN!

You Will Build Muscle and Lose Weight

Muscle mass begins to decline about 1 percent a year from the age of 30, and it accelerates after the age of 45. This creates a problem for fortysomethings, because as your muscle falls away, your body's calorie-burning action—its metabolism—slows down. We're talking about your resting metabolism, the rate at which your body burns calories to perform its essential functions, like breathing and pumping blood and digesting the deep-dish pizza you had for dinner. If you eat the way you did in your twenties and thirties, when you had more calorie-burning muscle, you're going to put on weight. That's an indisputable fact. And that explains the preponderance of the population with excess belly fat.

But, once again, it doesn't have to be that way. Studies show that even the elderly can build muscle, increase strength, and ramp up their metabolisms—even into their 90s. For you, a mere youngster in this scenario, it means you can easily keep the weight off with the right combination of strength- and muscle-building exercises that you'll find in this book. Even if you never picked up a dumbbell in your life, it's not too late. In fact, building muscular strength is one of the most critical things you can do to ensure a healthy, lean, and active life at 40+. With a greater ratio of muscle to fat, your metabolism will rev higher, and you won't have to worry about counting calories. Your active tissue will take care of all that. How's that for good news?

You Will Look and Feel 10 Years Younger

It's not just the *quantity* of the muscle you lose that's important, but also the *quality*. Research shows that as you age, fast-twitch muscle fibers shrink twice as fast as slow-twitch fibers. Why should you care? Because your fast-twitch fibers are the muscles largely responsible for generating power, the key to peak sports performance when you're young, and getting your butt out of a chair when you're old, says Alex Koch, PhD, an exercise researcher at Truman State University. And everyone knows intuitively how muscles tighten with the passing years. When you reach down but still can't pick up the ball on the tennis court or find yourself stuck to the mat in a seated yoga pose, that's all due to your declining fast-twitch muscles. If you target these muscle fibers with the exercises we show you—and elongate your muscles with proper stretches—you'll actually put more spring in your step, and, yes, keep up with your teenagers on the basketball court.

Oh, and by the way: Unlike explosive muscular power, muscular endurance doesn't naturally abate as you reach your 40s; it actually improves, as long as you stay fit. So if you stay strong, and keep your muscle tone, you'll actually be a better athlete than your teens are—because you'll have greater endurance.

You Will Injury-Proof Your Body

Think of your skeletal system as your personal infrastructure. Like our nation's roads and bridges, your bones will weaken and fail without maintenance. Or they will turn brittle with age, a condition called osteoporosis. Although often considered a women's disease, osteoporosis, or "porous bones," affects plenty of men, too. Keep your bones healthy throughout your life by getting adequate amounts of calcium and vitamin D, a nutrient that helps calcium leave the intestine and enter the bloodstream, and by doing *strength- and muscle-building exercises.* (Starting to see a pattern here?) Weight lifting helps strengthen bone because it increases the weight of gravity on your frame. Brisk walking, rope jumping, and exercises you'll read about later stimulate cells to build more bone, particularly in your back and hips. But lifting weights in your 40s requires more care and specific exercises, which you'll find in these pages.

You Will Have More and Hotter Sex

The fitter the body, the better the sex. True for women *and* men. Exercise whips up the libido, lifts mood and energy levels, and improves blood flow to the genitals. One study found that women who cycled for 20 minutes before watching an erotic video experienced a greater level of sexual arousal than women who didn't pedal up to the DVD. And a wealth of research indicates that men who are fit enjoy firmer erections. One large study of 31,000 men found that guys over 50 who walked just 2 miles a day had half the rate of erection problems of more sedentary men. "The harder the erection, the healthier the man," says Steven Lamm, MD, author of *The Hardness Factor* and a faculty member at the New York University School of Medicine. "When a man's blood vessels are healthy and elastic, his heart and brain are functioning well—and his erections are rock hard."

You Will Live Longer

We all live without ever knowing when our day of reckoning will come. But there are a few things you can do to exert control over your lifespan, things that can dramatically improve your chances of spoiling your great-grandchildren. The first are just common sense: Buckle your seatbelt, and put away the cell phone while driving. But there are others nearly as simple.

➡ BREAK A SWEAT DAILY: "If you had to pick one thing to make people healthier as they age, it would be aerobic exercise," says James Fries, MD, senior author of a new study at the Stanford University School of Medicine on the effects of running on aging. The research tracked 538 runners over age 50 and compared them to a similar group of non-runners. It found that runners have fewer disabilities, have a longer span of active life, and are half as likely as non-runners to die early deaths. Nineteen years after the study began, 34 percent of the non-runners had died compared to only 15 percent of the runners. In addition, the runners' first disability occurred an average of 16 years later than the non-runners' disabilities. (Think about that: Choosing not to exercise in your 40s could set you up for 16 years of disability—disability that could have been avoided. That's why we call this *the crucial decade.*) "We didn't expect this," says Fries. "The health benefits of exercise are greater than we thought."

➡ **EAT SMART TO LIVE LONG:** We'll show you how to choose foods that activate your longevity genes and avoid those linked to the diseases of aging—cancer, heart disease, Alzheimer's, diabetes. Antioxidant-rich foods can protect your cells and forestall many diseases, as you'll read in Chapter 3. We'll also tell you how to make savvy choices about vitamins and supplements.

You Will Think Faster and Smarter

Everyone's memory starts to get a little misty right after college—and not just because of all the keg stands. Your gray matter shrinks with age, nearly 2 percent every 10 years starting in your twenties, and some memory loss is inevitable the older you get.

But neuroscientists are learning that the adult brain can still grow (a process they call neurogenesis). Brain scientists have found that the dendrites (branch-like projections on some neurons) that receive electrical signals from other neurons are physically malleable. This means that it may one day be possible to grow new cells to replace ones damaged by disease or spinal cord injury. But it also suggests that you can trigger the growth of new brain cells and help your brain rewire its circuits. How? By eating brain-enhancing foods (generally those that are good for your heart—fish, vegetables, fruit), challenging yourself mentally, and staying physically active.

"Every man over 40 should exercise vigorously every day, even if it's only for two minutes, " says John Ratey, MD, an associate clinical professor of psychiatry at Harvard Medical School and the author of *Spark: The Revolutionary New Science of Exercise and the Brain.* Exercise gives your brain a greater blood supply, which can shield gray matter from damage. "A high heart rate challenges the brain, focusing it to adapt and grow," says Ratey.

You Will Manage Stress Better

Think of exercise as free medication, Dr. Ratey says. Aerobic exercise, specifically, has been shown to alleviate anxiety, stress, and even attention deficit disorder, he says. "Even people who are overweight and who start exercising see improvements in mood and cognition in as little as 12 weeks."

One landmark study at the University of Texas Southwestern showed that moderately intense aerobic exercise was just as effective as antidepressant medication in treating moderate depression. In that study, 80 depressed people were placed into five groups. Two of the groups did moderately intense aerobics for 30 minutes 3 or 5 days a week. Two other groups did lower-intensity aerobics, and a fifth group did stretches. After 12 weeks, those who worked out intensely 3 or 5 days a week, reduced their depressive symptoms by nearly 50 percent—on par with what would be expected for an antidepressant medication, says study author Madhukar Trivedi, PhD, director of UT Southwestern's mood disorders research program. "The key is that the exercise has to be rigorous and sustained for 30 to 35 minutes," he says.

Strength training seems to benefit the mind just as well. In one study at the University of Alabama, older men who lifted weights 3 times a week for 6 months improved their mood and reduced feelings of confusion, tension, and anger.

Although just how exercise reduces symptoms of depression and anxiety isn't fully understood, researchers believe that workouts raise the levels of mood-enhancing neurotransmitters in the brain. What *is* clear is that exercise boosts self-confidence and improves your ability to cope with setbacks. Exercise can provide a distraction from obsessive thoughts, as well as opportunities for interaction with people, which can combat feelings of isolation. "The brain feeds on social interaction, so when you combine exercise with group interaction, you maximize your brain's growth potential," says Dr. Ratey.

chapter 1

YOU DON'T HAVE TO GET FAT

Prime Your Muscles to Grow at Any Age

EMEMBER THAT KID from senior class who always wore the Smiths T-shirt and the skinny black jeans? Or the center on the basketball team who was so painfully thin that the lunchroom ladies gave him free seconds out of pity? Or how about the varsity cheerleader with the incredible long legs who was so nice (and hot) that even the mean girls treated her with respect? Now, see if you can find them at your 20th high school reunion. If it weren't for the name tags, you wouldn't know them. They've filled out, to put it nicely, but in reality they kind of look like Weebles. The changes in their bodies tell a simple human story. We all like to eat and drink. Pass the wings, please, and, sure, another beer with that.

Metabolism slows with the passing decades; we burn fewer calories in our 40s than we did in our 20s. Those are the facts. Here's another: *You don't have to gain weight as you age!*

Weight gain only seems like part of aging because so many➡

people in this XXL country of ours are overweight. But we're not talking about death and taxes here, inevitable parts of your future. You have control over your weight. You can press the stop button. You can be a skinny kid again—or pretty darn close. This book will show you exactly how. But to understand how to be lean, you have to first understand why so many of us get fat.

Our Bodies Burn Fewer Calories, But We Eat More

Healthy, active men in their 20s have about 13 to 17 percent body fat. By age 60, body fat composition rises, on average, to 19 to 26 percent. Why do our body compositions change this way? It happens because our muscle mass begins to decline by 1 to 2 percent a year from the age of 30 on, according to Roger Fielding, PhD, director of the Nutrition, Exercise Physiology, and Sarcopenia Laboratory at Tufts University's Jean Mayer USDA Human Nutrition Research Center on Aging.

Hold on a second. "Sarcopenia Laboratory?" What's that?

Sarcopenia is the scientific term for age-related muscle loss, the slow steady process that's very hard to detect because muscle is usually replaced by fat that infiltrates the tissue. A study in the *American Journal of Clinical Nutrition* found that for every pound of muscle a person loses, he or she will typically gain a pound of fat. Fortunately, new research indicates that you can stall and even reverse sarcopenia through strength training. Fielding's lab found that people who embarked on a program of moderate resistance training for about 30 minutes, five days a week, stopped the decline and added lean muscle tissue.

In another study conducted at East Tennessee State University, researchers studied 43 healthy people over age 55. Twenty-three of them did only aerobic exercise on a treadmill or stationary cycle. The other 20 subjects performed 15 minutes of aerobic exercise, then switched to training their major muscle groups on weight machines. After four months, the group that did strength training plus aerobics workouts significantly increased their lean muscle mass and bone density while the aerobics-only group saw no muscular improvement.

If you don't hold onto your skeletal muscle, your body will require fewer and fewer calories to function. (We're talking about your BMR here, your Basal Metabolic Rate, the amount of calories your body requires to breathe and pump blood and do all those other automatic life functions.) If your BMR declines, even if you don't increase your food consumption, you'll still put on weight.

Unfortunately, many of us don't curb our intake as we age, but instead increase the amount of food we eat. Why? As our disposable income grows, we tend to frequent restaurants a bit more. Our social calendars become full of opportunities to drink better wine and single-malt scotch, and fill up on artisan cheeses and those tasty little appetizers made of phyllo dough. Our kids' hunger for Happy Meals and chips and soda and ice cream influences our own snacking. And American food culture has super-sized our plates.

More unhealthy food available in larger quantities makes it easier for us to consume more. One study found that eating meals at restaurants versus at home increases calorie consumption by 500 calories per day. In 7 days, those extra calories would amount to 3,500 calories, the equivalent of 1 pound of additional weight. It's easy to see how quickly fat can happen when you consider that a typical muffin that weighed 1.5 ounces in 1957 has grown to 8 ounces and 400 calories today. A large soda back in the 1950s filled an 8-ounce cup. Today, the norm is 20 or more ounces and 200 to 400 calories. The average American's calorie consumption has jumped more than 10 percent since the 1970s. No wonder, then, that today the average man and woman weigh 191 and 140 pounds, respectively, roughly 24 more pounds each than they did in 1960.

We're Addicted to Sugar

Not only are we eating more food, but we are also eating more starchy carbohydrates such as processed grains, potatoes, corn, white rice, and sugar. Unlike protein, fat, and fiber—which have little if any impact on blood sugar—these "simple carbs" quickly break down and cause a fast increase in blood-sugar levels.

Today the average American consumes about 154 pounds of added sugars per year, about 45 pounds more than we ate in the 1950s. Most of this increase comes from corn-sweetener additives. In the 1970s, food manufacturers started adding sugar to foods in the form of high-fructose corn syrup because it's cheap to produce and makes for highly profitable products. You'll find it in candy, cookies, cakes, juices, breads, condiments, frozen dinners, cereals, and soft drinks.

Soft drinks are the leading source of calories in the average American's diet, accounting for nearly one in every 10 calories consumed, according to a 2005 study. That's easy to understand when you consider that a 12-ounce can of soda contains about 13 teaspoons of sugar.

Fruit juice is no better than soda, and it may even be worse. It sounds natural and healthy, so you rationalize drinking more of it. And a typical bottle of pure juice contains 2 to 2.5 servings. Do you ever drink just half of the bottle? Of course not. But do you realize you're getting double the number of calories listed in the Nutrition Facts when you drink it all?

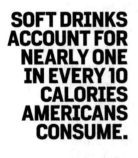

SOFT DRINKS ACCOUNT FOR NEARLY ONE IN EVERY 10 CALORIES AMERICANS CONSUME.

Sugary soft drinks are dangerous because your body perceives the calories in, say, a can of Pepsi as less filling than the calories in a medium apple slathered with a tablespoon of chunky peanut butter even though both are 165 calories. In a study at Purdue University, researchers gave subjects foods in both liquid and solid forms on different days of the week. It turned out that the people consumed many more calories on the days when they drank their meals compared with when they ate solid food.

This is one reason why eating whole fruit instead of drinking fruit juice is a smarter choice. The skin and pulp of a solid fruit (like apples and pears) contain fiber, which slows down the sugar infusion into your blood because it takes time to break down the fiber through digestion. A 2007 study in the *International*

Journal of Obesity reported that people who substituted a piece of whole fruit for fruit juice with their lunch reduced their daily calories by as much as 20 percent. Making that simple behavioral change in your diet could do wonders for your waistline.

While our consumption of sugary drinks has skyrocketed, so has our consumption of refined grains and cereal products. The sugars from these "white" processed foods—breads, cakes, cookies, pastas, breakfast cereals—are absorbed into our bloodstream lightening fast, causing blood sugar to spike. To understand how this leads to weight gain, and possibly obesity and diabetes, it helps to review how our bodies break down food for fuel.

When you eat, say, a big serving of spaghetti or half a box of cookies, the fast-absorbing glucose floods your bloodstream quickly, essentially overloading your system with much more energy than it can deal with. So, your pancreas produces insulin to help save the day. The insulin ushers the surplus glucose over to your liver, where it is turned into glycogen and later stored in your body's fat cells as triglycerides. Insulin also dials your blood sugar way down, causing you to crave more starches. Indulge your yearning for a second helping of Fettuccine Alfredo or more Thin Mints, Do-si-dos, or Caramel Delights, and the process repeats: Blood sugar rises, insulin comes to the rescue, blood sugar dives, cravings soar, and so on. Over time, it will take much more insulin to do the same job that a little bit of insulin did before. This is called insulin resistance, and it's a marker of a disorder known as metabolic syndrome or prediabetes.

An alarming 54 million Americans are living with prediabetes, according to the U.S. Government's Centers for Disease Control and Prevention. Prediabetes is associated with every major age-related illness, including erectile dysfunction, blindness, kidney failure, cancer, and heart disease. Untreated, prediabetes will turn into full-blown type 2 diabetes, which doubles your risk of a heart attack. Other markers of metabolic syndrome are low HDL (the "good" cholesterol), high triglycerides (a blood fat), having a waist that's 40 inches or larger, and obesity, a condition so prevalent in the United States that last year it overtook smoking as the number one cause of premature heart attacks.

What's Your Risk?

You can ballpark your risk for prediabetes and heart disease with a simple test using a cloth tape measure. Take off your shirt and unbutton your pants so that no clothing restricts your belly. Wrap a cloth measuring tape around your abdomen so that the bottom edge of the tape touches the tops of your hipbones. Do this in front of a mirror to make sure the tape isn't angled; it should be parallel with the floor. Stand straight and exhale, letting your belly relax as you pull the tape taught against the skin. (Don't compress the skin with the tape.) Look at the number corresponding with the "0" on the tape. That is the measurement of your waist. A waist size of 40 or more inches (35 or more for women), indicates that you are at high risk for metabolic syndrome.

Another way to check your health is to use the Body Mass Index, or BMI, which measures your body fat content based on your height and weight. The easiest way to find your BMI is to plug in your height and weight at an online BMI calculator, such as the one found at www.nhlbisupport.com/bmi/. Or check the BMI chart on the facing page.

How to Keep Pounds off at 40+

Okay, so now you understand why aging demands a smarter diet. Our muscle/fat composition changes, slowing the rate at which we burn calories. But our eating doesn't slow along with it, and as a result we continue to overload our plates with the kinds of foods that are making Americans overweight and dangerously unhealthy. What are you going to do about it? The answer is easy: Take in fewer calories, and learn to boost your metabolic burn. Accomplishing that is a lot tougher than it sounds because you're dealing with long-established eating patterns, an addiction to fast-absorbing carbohydrates, and a culture where working almost always means sitting. But if you can just begin, the results can be amazing.

Let's play around with some rough numbers. Due to the natural decline in basal metabolic rate that is associated with aging, a forty-something man weighing 180 pounds probably burns

Find Your Body Mass Index

For a quick measure of your health risk from too much body weight, use the Body Mass Index (or BMI) chart below

Look for your height in inches on the left side of the chart, then look to the right to find your weight. You'll discover your Body Mass Index at the very top of that column. Note that the BMI is just a rough estimate. Having more muscle on your frame will likely skew your BMI results, elevating you into the overweight or even obese zone when you may be perfectly normal. You can get a more accurate measure of body fatness by asking a nutritionist or trainer at your gym to give you a skin-fold thickness check with calipers.

BMI (kg/m²)	21	22	23	24	25	26	27	28	29	30	35	40	41	42
HEIGHT (in.)						WEIGHT (lb.)								
58	100	105	110	115	119	124	129	134	138	143	167	191	196	201
59	104	109	114	119	124	128	133	138	143	148	173	198	203	208
60	107	112	118	123	128	133	138	143	148	153	179	204	209	215
61	111	116	122	127	132	137	143	148	153	158	185	211	217	222
62	115	120	126	131	136	142	147	153	158	164	191	218	224	229
63	118	124	130	135	141	146	152	158	163	169	197	225	231	237
64	122	128	134	140	145	151	157	163	169	174	204	232	238	244
65	126	132	138	144	150	156	162	168	174	180	210	240	246	252
66	130	136	142	148	155	161	167	173	179	186	216	247	253	260
67	134	140	146	153	159	166	172	178	185	191	223	255	261	268
68	138	144	151	158	164	171	177	184	190	197	230	262	269	276
69	142	149	155	162	169	176	182	189	196	203	236	270	277	284
70	146	153	160	167	174	181	188	195	202	207	243	278	285	292
71	150	157	165	172	179	186	193	200	208	215	250	286	293	301
72	154	162	169	177	184	191	199	206	213	221	258	294	302	309
73	159	166	174	182	189	197	204	212	219	227	265	302	310	318
74	163	171	179	186	194	202	210	218	225	233	272	311	319	326
75	168	176	184	192	200	208	216	224	232	240	279	319	327	335
76	172	180	189	197	205	213	221	230	238	246	287	328	336	344

BMI CHART KEY: *Normal: 18-24* **Overweight:** *25-29* **Obese:** *30-39* **Extremely obese:** *40 and above*
Find an expanded BMI table at www.nhlbi.nih.gov/guidelines/obesity/bmi_tbl.pdf

250 or fewer calories per day than he did in his 20s. Figure he's in a desk job where he sits six or seven hours a day. (Australian researchers found that people who log more than 6 hours of chair time a day are 68 percent more likely to be overweight than those who sit for less time.) When you sit, you burn 1 calorie less per minute than when you stand. That's 420 calories you're not burning in 7 hours of sitting at your computer. Okay, now maybe it's your habit to order a mocha latte with whipped cream every morning (510 calories) and swig a Red Bull Energy Drink (160 calories) for an afternoon pick-me-up.

$$250 + 420 + 670 = 1340$$

That's a 1340-calorie difference from age 18, when "work" meant waiting tables or mowing the lawns of sedentary retirees, and you couldn't afford such decadent coffee drinks (or more to the point, the damn things hadn't been invented yet). That's more than a pound and half's worth of calories in five workdays. No wonder a study found that the typical office worker puts on 16 pounds in the first 8 months of a sit-down office job.

But here's how easily you can trim back on those extra calories. Cut out a few high-calorie drinks a day, and you'll be 670 calories better off. Stand at your computer for four hours of the day and take a walk after lunch, and you can eliminate those 420 sedentary calories. Now all you have to deal with is the 250 extra calories you've been given by your lethargic metabolism. Suddenly, things don't seem so daunting. And starting an exercise plan seems to be a pretty good idea.

Prime Your Muscles to Grow and Burn

Muscles are one of the biggest consumers of calories. As we mentioned earlier, when you get into your 40s, you start to lose muscle cells and your muscle fibers decrease in size. A study in the *American Journal of Clinical Nutrition* found that for every pound of muscle a person loses, he or she will typically gain a pound of fat. And sedentary people may lose 15 percent or more of their muscle mass each decade. If you lost 6 pounds of muscle over time, it's likely you've replaced it with 6 pounds of fat. And because fat is not as metabolically active as muscle is—in other words, fat burns fewer calories than muscle does—that means your resting metabolic rate is slower. What's more, more fat will make you look larger even if your total bodyweight stays the same, because one pound of fat takes up 18 percent more space on your skeleton than a pound of muscle. Fat blows us up like party balloons.

But muscle—muscle keeps us looking lean. It's packed harder and it requires up to 50 more calories daily than fat does, simply to exist. Mold more muscle onto your frame, and you'll fry more fat even when you're chilling on the couch. What's more, the fat you incinerate will be the most damaging kind: intra-abdominal or visceral fat. Unlike subcutaneous fat that's found just below the skin, the visceral variety is found deep inside your body, surrounding your viscera (your organs). This type of fat secretes harmful substances that raise blood sugar, contribute to inflammation of the arteries (a heart-disease risk factor), and increase your risk for prediabetes.

Fortunately, you can plot a surgical strike on that dangerous fat with strength training and moderate aerobic exercise. In a Canadian study of 52 obese men, researchers found that losing just 11 percent of your body weight can result in a 4-percent reduction in visceral fat. Other research shows that by increasing the intensity of your physical activity you can experience even greater declines in this dangerous fat. In a study at Duke University Medical Center, researchers placed 170 subjects into one of four groups: no exercise, low dose/moderate intensity (12 miles of walking per week), low dose/vigorous intensity (12 miles of running per week) and high dose/vigorous intensity (20 miles of jogging per week). After six months of exercise, computed tomography (CT) scans showed no change in fat in either of the low exercise groups but up to an 8 percent decrease in visceral fat for the group that exercised the hardest.

Strength training with weights appears to directly fight abdominal fat, according to a study of overweight people funded by the National Institutes of Health and conducted at the University of Pennsylvania in 2006. Compared to participants who received only advice about exercise, those given an hour of weight training twice a week reduced their proportion of body fat by 4 percent and were more successful in keeping off visceral fat. Strength training is a time-efficient way to prevent weight gain for adults, says study author Kathryn Schmitz, PhD, assistant professor at the Center for Clinical Epidemiology and Biostatistics at the University of Pennsylvania.

Historically, the scientific and medical communities have taken muscle for granted, but that's changing. "We used to discourage older adults from lifting heavy weights," says Wojtek Chodzko-Zajko, PhD, a professor of kinesiology and community health at the University of Illinois. "Now we're telling them they can't maintain overall health without it. After age 50, you can't get by just doing aerobic exercise."

Not only are diminished muscle strength and mass empirically linked to the onset of heart disease and diabetes, they also play a role in weaker bones, stiffer joints, slumping postures, and immune system decline. New research is looking into the possibility of measurable correlations between diminished muscle mass and cancer mortality. And it has been observed that people with less muscle mass respond poorly to physical stress. A 2000 study examining lung-cancer patients undergoing chemotherapy showed that the recurrence of cancer was predicted by levels of body protein. A 2004 study in the *Annals of Medicine* demonstrated a clear link to cardiac failure. And a 2006 study in the *Journal of the American College of Surgeons* found that severe burn victims with reduced muscle mass were less likely to survive.

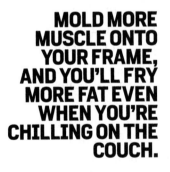

MOLD MORE MUSCLE ONTO YOUR FRAME, AND YOU'LL FRY MORE FAT EVEN WHEN YOU'RE CHILLING ON THE COUCH.

The increasing awareness about the role of muscle for good health is creating a major shift in the American preventive medical paradigm. Although it's not explicit yet in the government's overall health guidelines, agencies such as the Centers for Disease Control and Prevention now recommend a couple of rounds of resistance training a week. "Muscle function can improve—sometimes robustly—with resistance training, even after the onset of sarcopenia," says Robert Wolfe, PhD, a professor of geriatrics at the University of Arkansas for Medical Sciences. "But it is far more effective to begin resistance training before the process gains momentum. Intervention in the middle years is necessary."

Fire Up Your "Youth Muscles"

You have about 650 muscles attached to your bones, and each muscle is made up of bundles of muscle fibers. These skeletal muscles are called voluntary muscles because you control them when you flex your arm or kick a soccer ball. The other main kind of muscle is called smooth involuntary muscle, and it is found in the stomach and intestinal walls and in internal organs. You can't move these muscles no matter how hard you concentrate; they are controlled by the autonomic nervous system.

When we think of muscle, however, we're mostly thinking about the skeletal muscles, which attach to bones by tendons and get sore when you work with a shovel in the garden or lift weights. A lot of skeletal muscles act in pairs. The *flexor* muscles, such as the biceps, cause a joint to close. *Extensor* muscles, like the triceps, cause a joint to open. All of these skeletal muscles are signaled to contract by electrical impulses that travel from your spinal cord to muscle cells. A chemical neurotransmitter jumps the microscopic space between the nerve and the muscle cell, causing it to contract.

You have two main types of muscle fibers: type I, called slow twitch, and type II, called fast twitch, in roughly a 50:50 ratio on your skeleton. Slow-twitch muscles are the ones you use for extended periods of muscle contractions, like running a 10K. Since they twitch or fire more slowly, they are more efficient at using oxygen to generate muscle fuel (called adenosine triphosphate or ATP) and can go a long time before fatiguing.

Fast-twitch muscle fibers, by contrast, use an anaerobic ("without oxygen") system to generate energy. They fire rapidly, creating short, powerful bursts of speed, such as a sprint, or short-lived strength, like lifting a heavy weight or getting out of a beanbag chair. Because they have the highest rate of contraction and do so anaerobically, these muscles fatigue quickly. That's why you can't sprint very far or crank out a set of heavy squats without needing rest soon.

Why is it important to know about your different types of muscles? Because as we've already mentioned, when you get older your fast-twitch muscle fibers shrink more dramatically and quickly than your slow-twitch fibers do. (That's why they deserve the moniker "youth muscles," because the power of these fast-twitch muscles is what determines whether you perform like a 2nd-year quarterback ready to break into the starting lineup, or like a recently retired old pro hawking diet plans on ESPN.)

It's estimated that, over time, fast-twitch fibers lose half their size, compared to less than a quarter for slow-twitch fibers. For example, if your biceps consist of 90 fibers when you're 50 years old, by age 80 that number may be closer to 50 fibers and be made up of mostly slow-twitch. "This could be why older sprinters have up to 40 percent shorter stride lengths and need to take many more steps to cover the same distance as younger sprinters," says orthopedist Vonda Wright, who studies master's athletes. This decline in fast-twitch is significant even if you aren't an aging sprinter. Want to be able to make it to second base at next summer's annual softball marathon? Want to be nimble enough to dodge a killer taxi on Sixth Avenue? Then focus on muscle, especially the fast-twitch kind.

"Regular resistance is your most effective anti-aging weapon," declares Jeff Volek, PhD, RD, an exercise and diet researcher at the University of Connecticut. "Lifting weights signals your body to fight to keep your muscle."

Lest you think that your regular tennis game or swimming routine in a lap pool is enough, consider this research comparing three groups: masters athletes who did weight training in addition to running and swimming, masters athletes who did no weight lifting, and a group of same-age couch potatoes. The older athletes who did no strength training had a muscular composition similar to the sedentary people—even though they were in much better aerobic shape. However, the masters swimmers and runners who lifted weights regularly had muscle fiber composition similar to a control group 40 years younger!

Resistance Training — The Fountain of Youth

In Chapter 7, we've paired an ideal resistance training workout with a series of cardio interval workouts that will help you to get back in shape fast and stay that way with sports and exercise activities that you can do well into your 80s, even 90s. It's not just weightlifting that's crucial for healthy aging, but how you go about doing it. Fielding's research at Tufts shows that building power may be even more important than building strength. "Power has a velocity component to it," he says. "Often functional performance is dictated by how fast something can be done." He cites the example of someone who trips on a step. That person must make instant, rapid muscular adjustments to catch his balance to avoid falling. Speed of muscle movement is critical to saving you from a face plant on the pavement. And testing by Fielding's research group suggests that rapid weight lifting as opposed to the slow mode of traditional lifting may help maintain fast-twitch muscle power with age. Preliminary studies involving two groups of exercisers—one that did traditional slow lifting and another that did power training—found that muscle power output increased dramatically in the group that did the more explosive style of lifting. We incorporate that type of training into some of the strength-building exercises that we present later on in the book.

The beauty of these workouts is that they are versatile enough for almost anyone at any fitness level. If you're a sedentary beginner, you'll choose a more gradual and less intense path. People who are looking to lose that stubborn last 10 pounds or to up their training for, say, a triathlon competition will find something that targets their needs, too. The trick is developing the workout that fits your personality and goals and time commitment. Once you start losing weight and feeling great, the motivation will take care of itself.

For now, if you need more motivation to embrace a commitment to get back in shape for good, consider these additional benefits of strength training.

+ **You'll avoid tough breaks.** Recent research shows that strength training will strengthen your bones, reducing your risk of suffering a debilitating fracture in your hips or vertebrae. Plus, it improves your posture and alignment, so you don't turn into the Quasimodo of Snowbird Retirement Village when you're 83.

+ **You'll outrace diabetes.** Researchers at the University of Massachusetts found that men who added two total-body weight workouts a week to their existing aerobic exercise program had insulin levels that were 25 percent lower after a meal that was high in carbohydrates than the levels of men who performed the same aerobic exercise program but didn't lift weights. Another study found that you'll burn 73 percent more calories when you eat right after a workout.

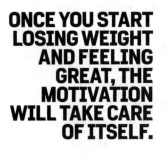

ONCE YOU START LOSING WEIGHT AND FEELING GREAT, THE MOTIVATION WILL TAKE CARE OF ITSELF.

You don't even have to work out very long to reap the benefits as long as you work out *hard*. A recent study at Heriot-Watt University in Edinburgh showed that high-intensity interval workouts lasting as little as three minutes may help prevent diabetes. In the study, out-of-shape men rode an exercise bike four to six times a day in rigorous 30-second bursts of speed, just twice a week. After 2 weeks, their insulin sensitivity improved 23 percent on average, and aerobic performance improved about 6 percent. "You can make just as big an effect doing short bouts of exercise as doing hours and hours of endurance training each week," says James Timmons, an exercise biologist who led the study. "Tense muscle contractions during sprints can really enhance insulin's ability to clear glucose out of the bloodstream."

+ **You may protect your brain.** Researchers at the University of Michigan found that people who performed three total-body weight workouts per week for 2 months lowered their blood-pressure readings by an average of eight points. That's enough to reduce the risk of a stroke by 40 percent.

+ **You'll be able to tie your own shoes at 95.** If you don't do anything to intervene, your flexibility will decrease by up to 50 percent between the ages of 30 and 70. Tight hip flexors can make it difficult to bend your knees enough to sit on the floor and then get back up again without the aid of a block and tackle. Poor range of motion in the shoulder joints will make it nearly impossible during the holidays to reach the brandy you've hidden on the top shelf in the cabinet. Regular stretching can help you avoid this, but so can weight training. A study in the *International Journal of Sports Medicine* showed that three total-body workouts a week for 16 weeks improved subjects' flexibility of the hips and shoulders by more than 30 percent and helped them better their sit-and-reach test scores by 11 percent.

Okay, then, are you ready to build some muscle and stay limber enough to reach those dumbbells at your feet? Good, but first grab a napkin. You need the right fuel to do the job. The next chapter will help you to think of food in a whole new way and establish some important habits of good nutrition.

chapter 2

THE GET-BACK-IN-SHAPE DIET

An Incredibly Simple Plan — 10 Foods You Should Eat Every Day

HEN HE WAS A MEDICAL STUDENT, Keith Block suffered from excruciating migraines and ulcers that left him doubled over. You would think that he was in a good place—medical school—to find a remedy. No deal. None of the physicians he visited provided any significant relief. Month after month, he tried to find a cure. Hypnotherapy, acupuncture, Rolfing massage, and more . . . nothing worked.

"Out of desperation, I stopped eating the roast beef, burgers, and fried chicken I'd been raised on, in favor of whole grains, legumes, and fruit," says the physician, now 55. "The idea that nutrition could help fight pain and illness was, in the medical community of the 1970s, unheard of. Yet within weeks, my ulcers and migraines disappeared."

Block's experience in med school changed his life and profoundly influenced his career. He is now the medical director of the Block Center for Integrative Cancer Treatment in Evanston, ➡

Illinois, where nutrition plays an important role in the individual-ized treatment plans developed for patients as well as people who are interested in the prevention of other diseases.

"There is a significant amount of research that shows that eating the wrong fats and proteins, primarily from animal sources, but also including omega-6-rich vegetables oils, can actually inflame cells and create a perfect environment for cancer, like a dry forest waiting for a spark," he explains. By contrast, diets based on plants and cold-water fish or omega-3 supplements lead to what he calls a "wet forest" that can affect the cells by reducing inflammation, a risk factor for not only cancer but also prediabetes and heart disease.

THE DECADE OF YOUR 40s IS A CRUCIAL TIME TO ESTABLISH A WET, GREEN FOREST WITHIN YOUR BODY.

The decade of your 40s is a crucial time to establish a wet, green forest within your body that will keep you healthier, leaner, younger-looking, and stronger for decades to come. How to start? First clean out your cabinets and refrigerator of processed foods, sodas, and juices, "white foods" like white bread and rice, cereals and baked goods, and make a major restocking trip to a supermarket with a robust produce section.

"At the grocery store, kale, tomatoes and [berries] won't have a single label touting their nutritional benefits," says Block, "but that's only because fresh produce doesn't have much of a mar-keting department."

As a guide, use the list of **10 Foods to Eat Every Day**, beginning on page 43. At the same time, begin practicing the following six critical eating principles that will help you to establish healthy habits for sustained weight loss and good health.

+6 STEPS FOR SMART EATING

HOW YOU EAT IS JUST AS IMPORTANT AS WHAT YOU EAT

1 EAT MORE OFTEN TO WEIGH LESS

Notice, we said "eat more often," not "eat more food." That's an important distinction because calories still count. You want to eat smaller meals, but more of them. This principle may sound counterintuitive, but it works brilliantly because it allows you to take optimal advantage of your body's most significant calorie-burning mechanisms: the thermic effect of eating and your basal metabolism. Your basal metabolism, also called your resting metabolism, reflects the calories that your body burns just through the normal course of living, even when you are plopped in front of the TV set, sleeping, or stuck in traffic. It's the total

calories it takes to keep your heart pumping, your brain daydreaming, and your lungs bellowing, and it makes up as much as 80 percent of your daily calorie burn.

Digesting food takes energy, too, up to 30 percent of your calories depending upon what you consume. That's because proteins require more energy to digest than do either fats or carbohydrates. If you think about it, the thermic effect of eating and your basal metabolism make up the vast majority of your body's calorie-burning capabilities, while exercising, walking to the refrigerator, and moving the sofa incinerate relatively few calories by comparison. By eating smaller meals more often during the day—at least four and as many as six to eight—you keep both mechanisms revving high.

Skipping meals throttles down your metabolism, reducing the effectiveness of the resting/digesting calorie burn. What's more, a stomach that's empty has an uncanny ability to make you ravenous, triggering your brain to send you hunting for the nearest food source—a box of Little Debbies?—or encourage you to overeat at lunch. Here's what a six-meal eating schedule might look like.

6:30 AM .... Breakfast
10:00 AM .... Snack
12:30 PM .... Lunch
3:30 PM .... Snack
7:00 PM .... Dinner
8:00 PM .... Snack (optional)

2 EAT BREAKFAST EVERY DAY

After 8 to 12 hours without food, your body needs to refuel. Skip breakfast, and you may reduce your metabolic rate by up to 10 percent, says sports nutritionist Leslie Bonci, RD, of the University of Pittsburgh Medical Center. Within a half-hour of waking up, have a breakfast of high-quality protein along with plenty of slow-digesting carbohydrates. Because your carbohydrate resources are low after an overnight fast, this is the time to refuel your tank. Plus, it's best to eat the bulk of your carbs early in the day so you have plenty of time to burn them. Just be sure that your carbohydrates for breakfast come from whole fruits and whole grains. If you can, try to make breakfast your biggest meal of the day, making dinner your smallest main meal of the day. We Americans are culturally conditioned to eat a big dinner, but that works against us. Eating too much at supper time can ignite your appetite and trigger uncontrollable hunger later on, causing you to overeat late at night.

3 DRINK 12 CUPS OF WATER PER DAY

Does that sound like a lot? Not when you consider that the 12 cups includes water you get from food and the other non-alcoholic liquids you consume during the day. Don't bother counting. Better to simply get into a routine: Drink a glass of water when you wake up, have liquids with breakfast and a glass of water with each subsequent meal and snack, plus one in between meals, and make sure you drink before, during and after exercise. That kind of routine will keep you well-hydrated and deliver the benefits of this key to good health, which include:

→ **WEIGHT LOSS.** Water replaces high-calorie drinks, sugary sodas, and fruit juices, and fills you up. Often, thirst signals are mistaken for hunger pangs.

→ **BETTER HEART HEALTH.** A study in the American Journal of Epidemiology found that people who drank at least five glasses of water a day were 41 percent less likely to die of a heart attack than those who drank two or fewer.

→ **A CLEAR HEAD.** Headache and fatigue are often triggered by dehydration.

→ **EXERCISE ENDURANCE AND PERFORMANCE.** Studies show that losing just 1 to 2 percent of your body weight in sweat can significantly affect your energy levels, reaction time, and athletic performance.

4 CHOOSE HEALTHY CARBOHYDRATES

Baked goods, microwave oven meals, canned pastas, cured meats, and other processed foods are full of salt and other flavor enhancers, chemical preservatives, and refined sugars such as high-fructose corn syrup and refined flour, which can spike your blood sugar. Plus, they are typically very high in calories and may contain dangerous trans fats.

5 GET MORE FIBER AND PROTEIN

Foods high in fiber help usher cholesterol out of your body, and they slow down digestion which keeps your blood sugar levels stable. Nutritionists recommend 25 to 35 grams of fiber each day, yet the average American is lucky if he gets half that amount. Fiber-rich foods are typically whole fruits, beans and legumes, vegetables and whole grains. Also, try to have some protein with every meal and snack. "People need to understand that they must ➡

5 Reasons Most Diets Don't Work

*Almost every failed dieting attempt can be traced
back to a handful of mistakes that sabotaged good intentions.
Here they are. Don't fall for these traps*

1

YOU STARVE YOURSELF

Puritanical sacrifice may make you feel better temporarily, but it won't do anything for your weight-loss efforts. Cutting too many calories, especially the ones you get from protein, shifts your body into starvation mode, and it will conserve calories rather than burn them. Also, diets of food denial tend to make your body cannibalize muscle for fuel. That's not what you want. In fact, it's counterproductive. More muscle means a faster metabolism and less body fat. Make sure you're getting at least 1,800 calories from a wide variety of foods and you're not cutting out protein.

2

YOU EAT TOO FAST

The dash out the door in the morning with bagel in hand and the half-hour speed lunch don't allow your brain any say in the matter of satiety. It takes 15 to 20 minutes for full-belly signals to reach the appetite center of your brain. If you speed-eat, you'll still feel hungry even though you've eaten enough—and tend to head back for seconds or thirds. Try to slow things down. Develop the habit of putting your fork down between bites or taking a sip of water after you chew and swallow. Talk to your spouse at dinner—hey, there's a concept! Anything you can do to prolong the meal will help you to listen to your body's messages that you are satisfied with what you've eaten.

3

YOU HAVEN'T VANQUISHED CARB CRAVINGS

Bread, cereals, white rice, potatoes, snack foods—you've tried to do without them, but you keep going back. The strategy of eliminating fast-absorbing carbohydrates is difficult to maintain if you don't replace those bad carbs with better carbs. Your body craves carbohydrates. So, give in by replacing the white stuff with fiber-rich carbs that will help control blood glucose and insulin levels. Make all your cereals whole-grain cereals.

Replace white bread with whole grain. Eat nuts instead of M&M's. Broccoli and cauliflower instead of potatoes. Whole fruit instead of juice.

YOU DON'T LIKE TO COOK

Eating healthy at restaurants is very difficult. So, if you're not a fan of home cooking, you've got problems. Restaurant portions are always too large, and you have little control over the ingredients used. One study found that people consume 500 more calories per day when they eat at restaurants compared to when they prepare their own meals at home. And those calories add up. Learning to like cooking, and becoming adept with knives, measuring cups, and saucepans, will give you a huge advantage in your quest to get fit. So, belly up to the stove (that's the large piece of equipment in your house underneath your popcorn maker, i.e., microwave oven). Grab a can opener and a pot, and thumb over to page 96 for a couple of simple, healthy, one-pot meals. That's a good place to start cooking your belly away.

YOU REWARD YOURSELF DISPROPORTIONATELY

A funny thing happens when you start exercising again and drop a few pounds. You feel pretty damn proud of yourself and believe you are worthy of a meat lover's pizza reward with a pitcher of beer. Sorry to be the bearer of bad news, but we humans tend to overestimate the number of calories we burn through exercise. Studies have shown that often people who start to exercise regularly will still gain weight because they scarf more calories than they burn off. The best way to keep from negating your workouts with overeating is to get religious about portion size and avoid high-calorie foods and drinks. The habits you develop in your 40s and the meal plans in this book will help you get there.

TOP 5 CANCER-CAUSING FOODS

+ Bacon
+ Corn chips
+ Crackers, cookies, muffins
+ Doughnuts
+ French fries
+ Hot dogs
+ Processed meats
+ Potato chips

get adequate protein for bone health and muscle maintenance," says Bonci, a sports nutritionist for the Pittsburgh Steelers, Penguins, Pirates and the University of Pittsburgh's athletic department. Women need 60 to 70 grams a day; men need a minimum of 80 grams a day. "Protein promotes satiety and keeps blood glucose stable so you'll feel more energetic during the day."

6 CONTROL YOUR PORTIONS

This is your most effective way of reducing calories and losing weight because you control what you put into your mouth. Unfortunately, we tend to eat what we are given at restaurants and have a penchant for cleaning our plates. "People use forks with tines long enough to take out their tonsils," says Bonci. "We use 16-ounce glasses for orange juice when a serving size is just 6 ounces, and pour our morning cereal into soup bowls. You can control portions just by using smaller plates and glasses."

Restaurants are the biggest violators of portion distortion. Thanks to super-sized entrees, we no longer understand what constitutes a proper serving size or realize how many calories foods contain. Consider the typical fast-food meal of a double cheeseburger, fries, large soda, and apple pie that packs upwards of 2,200 calories, roughly the amount of energy a 190-pound man would burn by running 15 miles. Knowing how many calories you need to eat each day can help improve your food awareness. To estimate how many calories you need to consume in order to maintain your weight, you need to do a little math using a formula called the Harris Benedict Equation to assess your BMR or basal metabolic rate.

Your basal metabolism, as you know, is the number of calories you'd burn if you stayed in bed all day—the calories used for essential bodily functioning. (See box on page 52 for calculating BMR and caloric need.)

+10 FOODS TO EAT EVERY DAY

FOR THOUSANDS OF YEARS, people ate basically the same thing every day—foods that were readily available and fresh: mostly plants, with some eggs, meats, fish. They didn't have microwave pizza bagels, Snickers bars, 64-ounce bottles of Mountain Dew, or 180 types of breakfast cereals to choose from. Eating wasn't easy—the deer often outran the spear—but it was simple, unlike today, where we are tempted with such enormous variety and a Starbucks on every street corner.

Suppose you simplified your pantry. Suppose you got rid of all the junk in your home and constructed your meals from a core mix of versatile and healthy foodstuffs. You wouldn't succumb to temptation, at least not in your home. The Oreos are long gone. You got rid of your stash of Butterfingers and fed the kids their last box of Kraft Sponge Bob Square Pants Shape Macaroni and Cheese.

You couldn't eat badly because you'd have no more *bad* food to eat—only the good stuff. What's the good stuff? Following are 10 types of foods to choose from every day—foods that provide high-quality protein to build muscles, healthy fats to promote brain and heart health, fiber-rich carbohydrates to deliver long-burning energy, and fruits and vegetables packed with anti-cancer and anti-cell-aging nutrients. Make these your food staples, the foundation of healthy meals. In the next chapter, you'll learn about other healthy foods to add variety to your culinary life.

1 BEANS OR LEGUMES

Good for muscle growth, brain function, heart health

This is a three-for-one deal. Each bean or legume provides slow-burning carbohydrates, dietary fiber, and protein, and the sheer number of varieties of beans makes them easy to incorporate into your diet every day. The perfect utility players for your pantry, beans are a nutritious foundation for any meal.

All beans are good for your heart, but none can boost your brainpower like **black beans.** That's because they're full of anthocyanins, antioxidant compounds that have been shown to improve brain function and fight cancer. A ½-cup serving provides 8 grams of protein and 7.5 grams of fiber and is low in calories and free of saturated fat.

Kidney beans, perfect for your favorite chili recipe, are protein-packed complex carbohydrates that stabilize glucose levels. They have more omega-3s than any other kind of bean. Kidney beans are also rich in thiamine, which protects memory and brain function. Researchers have linked a thiamine deficiency to Alzheimer's disease.

Navy beans contain potassium, which regulates blood pressure and normal heart contractions.

Chickpeas (garbanzo beans) are high in fiber, which helps stabilize blood sugar, lowering the risk of type 2 diabetes. They also crush cholesterol. In one study, people who ate a diet fortified with garbanzo beans slashed LDL cholesterol levels by almost 5 percent.

Lentils are the tasty staple of Indian cuisine. Known in India as dal, lentils are eaten at almost every meal, and India is the world's largest producer and consumer of these tiny disc-shaped legumes. Try to incorporate this superfood into your diet at least three times a week. They are *that* good for you. Lentils provide protein, cholesterol-lowering soluble fiber, iron, and B vitamins. In addition, lentils are rich in folate.

Beware of beans masquerading as health food: Baked beans are healthy at their core but they come drenched in sugary sauce that doesn't do

Halt the Salt

Studies show that we significantly underestimate our sodium intake at every meal. Use this scale to see how much you're getting from some of America's favorite foods

- 1 strip bacon:
  150 mg
- 1 cup cornflakes with skim milk:
  300 mg
- 2 handfuls potato chips:
  360 mg
- 2 tablespoons Italian dressing:
  500 mg
- Large french-fries:
  600 mg

- 2 pickle spears:
  700 mg
- 1 cup chicken noodle soup:
  775 mg
- 18 pretzel twists:
  1,100 mg
- ¼ pound cheeseburger:
  1,200 mg

(A healthy person's daily sodium intake should range between 1,500 and 2,300 mg per day.)

- Large glass tomato juice:
  1,300 mg
- 4 buffalo wings:
  1,400 mg
- 3 ounces blue cheese:
  1,550 mg
- 8 slices salami:
  1,800 mg
- 2 tablespoons soy sauce:
  2,000 mg

you any favors. Likewise, stay clear of refried beans as many are made with lard, a saturated fat.

EASY WAYS TO EAT MORE:

➡ **WRAP BLACK BEANS IN A BREAKFAST BURRITO.** Or try this Black Bean and Tomato Salsa: Dice 4 tomatoes, 1 onion, 3 cloves of garlic, 2 jalapeño chile peppers (wear plastic gloves when handling), 1 yellow bell pepper, and 1 mango. Mix in a can of black beans and garnish with ½ cup chopped cilantro and the juice of 2 limes.

➡ **KIDNEY BEANS ARE A TERRIFIC TOPPER FOR SALADS.** Toss them into soups or spaghetti sauce. Or find a simple recipe for Pasta e Fagioli in a good Italian cookbook.

➡ **EAT HUMMUS SPREAD.** Chickpeas are the main ingredient in hummus, a garlicky bean spread that's great on crackers or as a substitute for mayonnaise on sandwiches.

➡ **ADD COOKED LENTILS TO SALADS.** They are terrific side dishes to pork and chicken. Make a hearty lentil soup for a main meal; or, for a quick lunch, heat up canned lentil soup. (Make sure you buy low-sodium varieties when using canned lentil soup.)

2 BERRIES AND GRAPES OR APPLES, PEARS, ORANGES

Good for heart health, immunity boosting, cancer fighting, brain health

Unless you've been living under a rock, you've no doubt heard the call to eat more fruit, especially berries. In general, the darker the color of the fruit, the more healthful nutrients it contains. And remember, frozen berries are just as nutritious as fresh ones, so keep your freezer stocked with bags of berries for snacking on, tossing into smoothies, and topping on salads and cereals.

Host to more antioxidants than any other popular fruit, **blueberries** help prevent cancer, diabetes, and age-related memory changes (hence the nickname "brain berry"). One particular antioxidant, *pterostilbene*, which is similar to the resveratrol in grapes, can stimulate liver cells to better break down fat and cholesterol, according to USDA scientists. Blueberries are also rich in fiber and vitamins A and C and are known to fight inflammation, the key driver of many chronic diseases.

Cranberries: Only wild blueberries boast more antioxidants than cranberries. This berry can also be called a natural probiotic, enhancing good bacteria levels in the gut.

Strawberries, raspberries, and blackberries all contain ellagic acid and a large number of polyphenols, which inhibit tumor growth. These berries are loaded with fiber; you get 8 grams in just one cup of raspberries or blackberries.

Red grapes are anti-aging

What to Drink

Avoid the stealthy calories in sodas and juices by switching to minimally sweetened teas and seltzers

What you drink with your meals will have a huge impact on your bottom-line calorie intake. The number of liquid calories we consume has increased by 93 percent since 1965, to the tune of 222 extra calories a day, according to a new study in the journal *Obesity*.

Researchers estimate that sweetened beverages account for most of this increase. And fruit drinks are a big part of the problem: They are loaded with calories, and many are full of high-fructose corn syrup (HFCS), which can quickly add pounds. A study of 43,960 women published in the *Archives of Internal Medicine* demonstrates how insidious drinks with empty calories can be. Women who drank two or more 8-ounce fruit drinks containing HFCS were 31 percent more likely to develop diabetes than women who consumed just one fruit drink a month. And those who drank two sodas a day increased their diabetes risk 24 percent compared to those who had just one a month.

Diet soft drinks, grapefruit juice, and orange juice did not appear to increase risk. But that doesn't mean you should swallow buckets of OJ. Even 100 percent fruit juice is still high in calories. Grab an orange instead. You can get your vitamin C, plus fiber, by eating whole fruit. And when you do drink OJ and grapefruit juice, cut it with some water. You'll trim calories and still get enough vitamin C. Or, for a healthy carbonated alternative to soft drinks, mix 100 percent fruit juice (tart cherry, açai, and pomegranate juices are richest in natural antioxidants) with seltzer water to make a fruit spritzer.

"One of my favorite alternatives to water is Polar seltzer, a no-sugar, no-sweetener, calorie-free drink that contains carbonated water and fruit essence," says David L. Katz, MD, the director of the Prevention Research Center at Yale School of Medicine.

Another good choice is Honest Tea, a line of minimally sweetened teas with the added benefit of concentrated antioxidants. And there's always hot coffee or tea. Both have antioxidants, neither has calories, and the caffeine adds a modest calorie-burning boost to your metabolism.

candy. Not only do grapes protect against stroke and heart attack, these sweet juicy fruits contain compounds that may help keep your skin flexible and elastic. And new research at the University of California suggests that the resveratrol in red grapes may help prevent colon cancer.

EASY WAYS TO EAT MORE:

➡ **EAT THEM DRIED OR IN JAM.** Blueberries maintain most of their power no matter what form they come in. When you can't get blueberries, try açai powder. The Amazonian berry it's made from has even more antioxidants than the blueberry. Mix 2 tablespoons of açai powder into orange juice, smoothies, breakfast cereal, or yogurt.

3 BROCCOLI OR SPINACH

Good for sexual enhancement, muscle growth, stronger bones, better eyesight, heart health

Alternate eating a serving of broccoli and spinach every day, and you'll guarantee that you're getting the mother lode of the most powerful and essential plant-based nutrients for preventing the diseases of aging. Broccoli (and its brother cruciferous vegetables cauliflower, Brussels sprouts, and cabbage) contains abundant amounts of the antioxidant compound *sulforaphane*, which has been shown to prevent cancer and remove toxins from cells. Broccoli, or "trees," as our kids like to say, is also a good source of vitamin C, fiber, folate, and phytochemicals that have been associated with reduced rates of specific cancers in the lung, colon, and bladder.

It may be green and leafy, but spinach is also a formidable power food. This noted biceps builder is a rich source of plant-based omega-3s and folate, an extremely important nutrient; these help reduce the risk of heart disease, stroke, and osteoporosis. In combination with vitamin B12, folate may protect the brain against dementia. Researchers from Tufts and Boston universities observed subjects in the Framingham Heart Study and found those participants with high levels of homo-

How to Eat Before and After Exercise

An easily digested snack of carbohydrates will energize your workout. But don't overdo it. Eat a more substantial meal post-exercise, when your muscles need to recharge and repair

Drink plenty of water before, during, and after exercise. Your heart and body work much harder when you become dehydrated.

Within 30 minutes after exercise, consume a carbohydrate-rich food along with a little bit of protein: a multigrain sandwich made with lettuce, tomato, and slices of lean turkey, for example. That is the best way to replenish intramuscular energy stores. It will also keep you from getting so hungry that you reach for the potato chips when you get home.

If you have a habit of downing workout drinks, consider a cup of low-fat chocolate milk (1%). With carbohydrates, calcium, and protein, chocolate milk is the perfect post-exercise drink and a lot less expensive than bottled energy-replacement drinks

---

cysteine had nearly double the risk of developing Alzheimer's disease. High homocysteine is associated with low levels of folate and vitamins B6 and B12, leading researchers to speculate that getting more B vitamins may be protective. Finally, spinach is packed with lutein, a compound that fights age-related macular degeneration. If the salad bar doesn't have spinach, grab the romaine lettuce. It's a good substitute in a pinch.

EASY WAYS TO EAT MORE:

➡ **STOCK UP ON FROZEN BROCCOLI SPEARS AND FLORETS** to cover yourself for those times when the "fresh" broccoli in your crisper looks limp and brown. Keep florets on hand to top your salads; toss broccoli into stir-fry dishes; use it as a side with chicken; and sprinkle grated Parmesan cheese on top of steamed broccoli to add a bit of salty flavor. Use spinach as the base of your salads; add spinach to scrambled eggs; drape it over pizza; mix it with marinara sauce and then microwave for an instant dip.

4 LEAN PROTEIN (EGGS, POULTRY, FISH, BEEF, PORK)
Good for muscle growth and recovery, satiety, boosting metabolism

Go for 3 or 4 ounces of lean beef, turkey, chicken, or fish, plus an egg or two every day. Try to make fish your protein two to four times a week—it's brain food. A 4-ounce serving of wild salmon has approximately 2,000 milligrams of DHA and EPA, two key omega-3 fatty acids that serve as oil for the brain's hardware, says dietitian Joan Salge Blake, author of *Nutrition and You*. People with the highest blood levels of this nutrient have a 47 percent lower chance of developing dementia, according to a study published in the *Archives of Neurology*. Another study from the University of Pittsburgh found that people who scored high on EPA/DHA blood screens were happier, less impulsive, and more agreeable. Oily cold-water fish also has anti-inflammatory properties and helps protect against joint inflammation, blood clots, and heart arrhythmias.

Beef contains two key muscle-building nutrients: iron and zinc. And it may also help you to lose weight because it is rich in conjugated linoleic acid (CLA). In several studies, people who ate diets high in CLA ended up losing weight and maintaining more lean muscle compared with people who avoided meat.

You know that chicken and turkey are good protein choices, but consider the other white meat: pork. Per gram of protein, pork chops contain almost five times the selenium—an essential mineral that's linked to a lower risk of prostate cancer—of beef, and twice that of chicken. And Purdue researchers found that a 6-ounce serving daily helped people preserve their muscle while losing weight.

EXPERT ADVICE

Q. What's the biggest mistake people make when dining at restaurants?

"They ignore portion size. A trick I use when dining out is to ask for something light as soon as I sit down—gazpacho or ceviche, for example. That way, I'm not ravenous when the main course arrives. Both options are also low glycemic (i.e., digested slowly), so they won't spike blood sugar levels, which, in turn, can trigger food cravings and feelings of hunger. If I'm ordering a salad, I stick to non-diet, regular dressing. The fat-free varieties make up for their lack of flavor with extra sugar, which can lead to a similar spike in blood sugar. I also never deny myself dessert, especially if it's chocolate cake. I do, however, limit myself to three bites. It's just as satisfying as eating the whole thing, and I'll still respect myself in the morning."

— **ARTHUR AGATSTON, MD,** *cardiologist and author of The South Beach Diet*

EASY WAYS TO EAT MORE:

➡ **CATCH FISH IN A CAN.**
You probably don't need advice on eating more meat. Fish, that's another story. Since fish can be time consuming to buy and a hassle to prepare, stock up on canned sardines and jarred pickled herring to make it a little easier to sneak fish into your week. Both sardines and herring have high amounts of omega-3 fatty acids. And a single can of sardines delivers more calcium than a cup of whole milk (because you eat the bones.) If you can grill some salmon once a week and round out your quota with canned fish, you'll be doing just fine.

5 OATMEAL
Good for stimulating the brain, muscle growth, a healthy heart

Let's give oatmeal its props. ➡

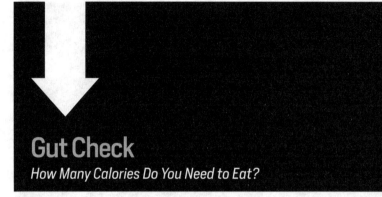

Gut Check
How Many Calories Do You Need to Eat?

Before you can lose weight through diet and exercise, it helps to know how many caloires your body requires to maintain it's current weight.

First, find your BMR. (Use an online BMR calculator, or do this math.)

→ **MEN** 66 + (6.2 x your weight in pounds) + (12.7 x your height in inches)—(6.8 x your age in years)

→ **WOMEN** 655 + (4.4 x your weight in pounds) + (4.7 x your height in inches) — (4.7 x your age in years)

THE HARRIS BENEDICT FORMULA To determine your total daily calorie needs based on your height, weight, age, and sex, multiply your BMR by the factor corresponding to your activity level.

If you are sedentary (little or no exercise):
→ **BMR** x **1.2**

If you are lightly active (light exercise or sports 1 to 3 days a week):
→ **BMR** x **1.375**

If you are moderately active (moderate exercise or sports 3 to 5 days per week):
→ **BMR** x **1.55**

If you are very active (hard exercise or sports 6 to 7 days per week):
→ **BMR** x **1.725**

If you are extra active (very hard exercise or sports and a physically demanding job):
→ **BMR** x **1.9**

So, for example, if you are a lightly active 43-year-old man who weighs 230 pounds and stands 5-feet-10-inches, you would multiply your BMR (2,089) by 1.375 = 2,872. This is the total number of calories you would need to maintain your current weight. If you want to lose weight, you would need to either consume less than 2,872 calories per day (calories in), or exercise

more (calories out), or a combination of both diet and exercise. A useful guideline for weight loss is to lower calorie intake by at least 200 calories per day while starting an exercise program.

Keeping track of calories is an effective weight-loss tool, but it's about as much fun as stripping old wallpaper. Use these simple portion-control guidelines to be more practical for daily use.

+ A serving of meat or fish is about the size of a deck of playing cards.
+ A serving of pasta is about the size of your fist. Same goes for potato or rice.
+ At a restaurant, cut your servings in half and ask the server to doggy-bag half of your meal before you begin eating.
+ When pouring yourself juice, use a juice glass (6 ounces), not a pint glass.

Not only is it a versatile and essential grain, it's so integral to good nutrition that it should be eaten nearly every morning, especially if you don't have the time to cook an omelet for yourself. Oatmeal will also fill you up with long-burning clean energy. Sure, oats are loaded with carbohydrates, but the release of those sugars is slowed by the fiber, and, because oats also have 10 grams of protein per ½-cup serving, they deliver steady muscle-building energy. In fact, studies show that oatmeal keeps insulin levels stable longer than most other foods, which means you won't find yourself sniffing around the home-baked cookies someone brought in to work an hour after you eat it.

There are two types of fiber: soluble fiber, which acts as a magnet for fluid and digests slower, and insoluble fiber, like that found in vegetables. Oatmeal has a lot of the soluble kind, which is why it has the reputation for clobbering cholesterol. Soluble fiber is believed to reduce your low-density lipoprotein (LDL), the "bad" cholesterol, by binding with digestive acids made from cholesterol and ushering them out of your body. This limits the absorption of cholesterol in your intestines. Ten grams or more of soluble fiber a day can decrease your total and LDL cholesterol. You have a couple of choices when it comes to oatmeal. Steel-cut oats contain more fiber: 2 or 3 grams more, for a total of 8 grams. The oats are chopped with steel blades, resulting in chewier oatmeal that's less processed than rolled oats. They'll keep you fuller longer, but they take longer to prepare. If you are pressed for time, the instant oatmeal (rolled oats) is a lot more convenient. But choose the unsweetened, unflavored variety to avoid tons of sugar. Instead, sweeten your oatmeal with berries, raisins, milk, nuts and a bit of honey.

EASY WAYS TO EAT MORE:
➡ **OATS AREN'T JUST FOR BREAKFAST.** You can incorporate them into other meals for a nutritional boost. Sprinkle oats in yogurt, bake them into cookies, or mix ¾ cup of uncooked oats with a pound of turkey breast, ½ cup of fat-free plain yogurt and ¼ cup

SMALL CHANGES, BIG RESULTS

Drink from a tall, narrow glass, and save yourself calories and a hangover. Our brains estimate height and width differently. Studies show that, given drinking glasses with the same capacity, subjects regularly pour more liquid into short, squat glasses than they do into tall, narrow ones.

chopped onion for fiber-rich turkey burgers.

Uncooked quick oats can also be used in an egg mixture to coat baked chicken.

6 OLIVE OIL OR AVOCADO

Antioxidant properties fight free-radical damage.
Good for cognitive function, healthy arteries

Olive oil may have a "wimpy" name, but it's a powerhouse food that controls cravings, helps burn fat, and can even build muscle. Olive oil is a monounsaturated fat that has been associated with everything from lower rates of heart disease and colon cancer to a reduced risk of diabetes and osteoporosis. You've heard about that for years. But it also appears that olive oil prevents muscle breakdown by lower-ing levels of a cellular protein that is linked to muscle wasting and weakness.

➡ **TIP:** Choose the extra-virgin olive oil, which has higher levels of the antioxidant vitamin E.

Avocado is also loaded with satiating, heart-healthy monounsaturated fat. It's been shown to improve blood flow to the brain, leading to better cognitive function. And the oleic acid in avocado lowers blood cholesterol.

7 PROBIOTIC YOGURT, LOW-FAT CHEESE, OR FAT-FREE MILK

Good for fighting cancer, strengthening bones, boosting immune system

Various cultures claim yogurt as their own creation, but this 2,000-year-old food's health benefits are not disputed:

Fermentation spawns hundreds of millions of probiotic organisms that serve as reinforcements to the battalions of beneficial bacteria in your gut, boosting the immune system and providing protection against cancer.

Not all yogurts are equal. You want the *probiotic* kind, so make sure the label says "live and active cultures." Another reason to eat yogurt: It is one of the few foods that contain conjugated linoleic acid, a special type of fat that some studies show can reduce body fat.

Aim for 1 cup a day of this calcium, carbohydrate, and protein-rich stuff.

EASY WAYS TO EAT MORE:

➡ **YOGURT TOPPED WITH BLUEBERRIES, WALNUTS, FLAXSEED, AND HONEY IS THE ULTIMATE BREAKFAST—OR DESSERT.** Plain low-fat yogurt is also a perfect base for creamy salad dressings and dips. Use in place of sour cream.

For variety, try Greek yogurt. Called yiaourti in Greece, this is a thicker, creamier yogurt because the liquid (whey) has been strained away. This rich yogurt contains probiotic cultures and has twice the protein of regular yogurt and fewer carbohydrates, and it is lower in lactose. Add chopped apples, pears and peaches, or berries and walnuts. The thick stuff will stand up to big chunks of fruit and nuts.

➡ **TRY THIS EASY HEALTH SMOOTHIE THAT PACKS A TON OF NUTRIENTS:** Blend 1 cup low-fat yogurt, 1 cup fresh or frozen blueberries, 1 cup carrot juice, and 1 cup fresh baby spinach.

➡ **DRINK MORE MILK.** Unless you're pouring it on your cereal or in your coffee, you probably don't pay much attention to milk. And that's a mistake because drinking a glass of milk is an easy way to get bone-building calcium, which has been shown to be crucial for weight loss.

A University of Tennessee study found that dieters who consumed three or more servings of calcium-rich foods a day lost nearly twice as much weight as those taking in less calcium. Researchers think the calcium from milk and other dairy foods probably prevents weight gain by increasing the breakdown ➡

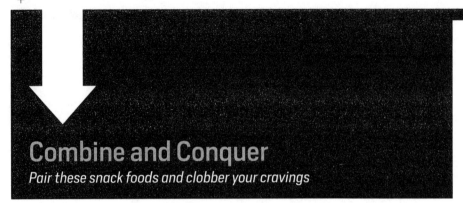

Combine and Conquer

Pair these snack foods and clobber your cravings

Snacking is one of the most powerful weight-loss tools in your arsenal. If you do it right, you'll avoid the fast drop in blood sugar that sends you hunting for cupcakes on the party table at work. Problem is that nobody ever taught us how to snack properly. Snacking means snack foods to red-blooded Americans. Little Debbies, Lay's Potato Chips, Slim Jims—heck, most anything you can get in the company vending machine.

Smart snacking involves some thought and preparation. Unless you have a good cafeteria at work that stays open past 3, you'll have to bring your snacks with you. The key is to plan ahead. For the most appetite-satisfying snacks, snacks that will keep hunger away for hours, combine something full of slow-absorbing carbohydrates with something rich in protein, and with a little fat.

See what delicious combinations you can come up with, and keep them on hand. Mix and match from columns 1 and 2.

COLUMN 1 **CARBS**	COLUMN 2 **PROTEIN/FAT**
Celery sticks	1 Tablespoon Reduced-fat cream cheese spread
4 dates	7 almonds
4 whole-wheat crackers	Whey protein drink
5 strawberries	1 cup low-fat yogurt
Raw baby carrots	2 Tablespoons hummus
1 medium apple	1 tablespoon peanut butter
¼ cup trail mix	1 cup 1% or low-fat chocolate milk
Whole-wheat tortilla	2 slices turkey breast and slice of Swiss cheese
1 pear	1 stick low-fat string cheese
1 cup berries	1 inch square hard cheese

of body fat and hampering its formation. Avoid the full-fat whole milk and drink fat-free or low-fat milk. You can wean yourself off the full-fat variety by mixing it with 2% or 1% milk and gradually using less and less of the whole milk.

8 TOMATOES OR RED/ YELLOW PEPPERS

Good for preventing cancer, boosting immunity, heart health

Here's what gives us the authority to call pizza a health food: tomatoes and tomato sauce. According to the FDA, eating tomatoes and tomato products may reduce the risk of prostate, gastric, and pancreatic cancers, thanks to their high concentration of the nutrient lycopene. This antioxidant can also reduce the risk of coronary artery disease. And processed tomatoes in pastes used for pasta and pizza sauces are just as potent as fresh whole tomatoes because they make it easier for the body to absorb the lycopene.

As for the bell peppers, red, yellow, green or orange are all good sources of vitamin C, vitamin B6, folic acid, and phytochemicals that ward off heart disease, stroke and cataracts.

EASY WAYS TO EAT MORE:
➡ **TOP YOUR SALAD WITH 8 RED CHERRY TOMATOES** and chopped yellow peppers. Drink a glass of low-sodium tomato juice instead of a soda. Double the amount of tomato paste called for in a recipe, and order double the tomato sauce on a take-out pizza pie. Bring sliced red peppers to work as a snack; they are so sweet they don't need dip. You can also get your lycopene and vitamin C from slices of watermelon, papaya and pink grapefruit.

9 NUTS OR PEANUT BUTTER

Good for heart health, brain function, protection from cell damage

Nuts are heart candy. In a study of more than 3,000 African American men and women, those who ate nuts at least five times a week cut their risk of dying of heart disease by 44 percent compared with people who ate nuts less frequently.

Most nuts are the perfect snack food, packed with

57

muscle-building protein, filling fiber, and heart-healthy monounsaturated fats, but two of the absolute best are walnuts and almonds.

Walnuts are one of the richest sources of alpha-linolenic acid (ALA), the plant-based omega-3 fatty acid, and have a positive effect on arteries, decreasing inflammation and reducing levels of substances that promote clogging. Almonds are full of fiber and a nutrient you probably never heard of, alpha-tocopherol, a form of vitamin E that reduces the risk of Alzheimer's disease, according to a National Institute on Aging study.

Walnuts, almonds, and other nuts also reduce levels of LDL cholesterol and of a compound called lipo-protein(a) that increases clotting and can lead to a stroke, according to a study published in *Annals of Internal Medicine*. But don't stop there; other nuts offer plenty of other health benefits.

Pistachios contain a plant cholesterol that can produce a 10-point drop in your triglycerides and a 16-point decline in your LDL cholesterol,

according to a report in the *Journal of the American College of Nutrition.*

Brazil nuts are richer in selenium than any other food. Selenium is a mineral that has been linked to preventing cancers of the prostate and colon.

Pecans deliver the most antioxidants of any nut. Adding them to your diet may reduce your risk of cancer, heart disease, and Alzheimer's disease. Just don't eat them in the pie.

EASY WAYS TO EAT MORE:

➡ **TOSS NUTS INTO SALADS.** Add them to baked goods. Top pancakes with walnuts. Spoon peanut butter into curries. Grind and mix nuts with olive oil to make a marinade for grilled fish or chicken. And keep a bag of mixed nuts in your work desk for snacking.

10 WHOLE GRAIN BREAD OR PASTA

Good for brain function, energy, controlling blood sugar and insulin levels

The brain is a furnace that requires a constant supply of fuel (in the form of glucose)

to perform. Fiber-rich whole grain foods, like whole grain bread, brown rice, and whole grain pasta, provide an even flow of glucose, and their B vitamins nourish the nervous system. University of Toronto researchers recently determined that eating carbohydrate-rich foods like whole grain bread is equivalent to a shot of glucose injected into your brain. According to the study, the higher the concentration of glucose in your blood, the better your memory and concentration.

EASY WAYS TO EAT MORE:

➡ **CALL IN THE REPLACEMENTS.** Judging from the number of sandwiches, pasta salads, and spaghetti dinners we eat, it's not going to be hard to eat more bread and pasta. It's the type we need to change. Do a clean sweep of your kitchen, tossing out all refined white breads, pastas, and rice, and highly processed cereals, and replacing them with whole grain bread, pasta, and brown rice. Make a habit of going whole grain all the time.

✚ BEVERAGES: GREEN TEA OR TART CHERRY JUICE

The antioxidant catechin, found in tea, promotes blood flow, which boosts brainpower by enhancing memory, mood, and focus. Green tea also boasts powerful anti-inflammatory properties.

Tart cherry juice is another potent source of antioxidants. Cherry juice has been used by traditional healers for hundreds of years as a folk remedy for gout because it lowers uric acid levels. Today, studies suggest that tart cherries and their juice are rich in plant compounds called anthocyanins that have strong anti-inflammatory effects and may protect neurons from oxidative damage.

Anthocyanins are known to inhibit cox-1 and cox-2 enzymes, which are involved in the production of prostaglandins, compounds that trigger inflammation. Sweet cherries have anthocyanins, too, but tart cherries have much higher concentrations, and they are a bit lower in sugar. You can buy tart cherry juice in bottle or concentrate form. Mix with seltzer for a refreshing, low-calorie, antioxidant-rich drink.

+HOW TO EAT AT 40+

A NEW 7-DAY HEALTHY-EATING PLAN YOU CAN LIVE WITH

YOU HAVE THE LIST. Now put it to good use. Using those 10 core foodstuffs described on the previous pages as your foundation, you can craft a full week of delicious eating that won't leave you with hunger pangs. To make it even easier, we've suggested seven breakfasts, lunches, dinners and snacks to start off with on the following pages. You don't even have think much about it. Just read and eat. Give these meals a try for a week or two, and then build upon your staples using the expanded shopping list of 40+ power foods in the next chapter. Within a week, you'll start to establish healthier eating habits that are easy to sustain because they're logical and delicious.

BREAKFAST

The morning meal means "breaking the fast." You've been fasting for the past 8 to 12 hours, mostly while asleep. Your metabolism has throttled down low, and now your brain and muscles crave a healthy dose of high-quality protein and slow-burning carbohydrates. Now is your best chance of the day to fuel up with food that will keep you feeling full longer, help you avoid midmorning cravings for croissants, and power your body for action.

Numerous studies back up what grandma's been saying for decades: Eat your breakfast. Researchers at Virginia

Commonwealth University found that dieters who regularly ate a protein-rich full breakfast lost significantly more weight (and kept it off longer) than another group that ate a low-cal breakfast with a quarter of the protein.

A study at the University of Kansas Medical Center and Purdue University showed that eating more protein for breakfast helps men avoid overeating the rest of the day. And other studies show that eating breakfast away from home (which typically involves pancakes) boosts your obesity risk by 137 percent, and skipping breakfast completely lifts your risk of becoming obese by 450 percent.

The ideal breakfast is high in protein (to keep you satiated), low in starch (to prevent swings in blood sugar), and packed with fiber-rich vegetables and whole grains to keep your mind sharp all morning long.

BREAKFAST #1

+ 1 whole egg and 2 egg whites scrambled in olive oil with ½ cup baby spinach
+ ½ cup oatmeal with blueberries
+ 1 cup green tea

Makes 1 serving. Per serving: 253 calories, 17 g protein, 21 g carbohydrates, 10 g fat (2 g saturated), 3 g fiber

BREAKFAST #2

+ 1 cup oatmeal with cinnamon and a handful of walnuts
+ ½ glass orange juice
+ 1 medium pear
+ 1 cup green tea or coffee (sweetened with calorie-free Splenda)

Makes 1 serving. Per serving: 514 calories, 13 g protein, 68 g carbohydrates, 24 g fat (2 g saturated), 12 g fiber

BREAKFAST #3

+ Green Eggs and Ham Cups (recipe on page 92) made with 2 eggs; ½ cup fresh spinach; 2 mushrooms, sliced; 2 tablespoons shredded reduced-fat Cheddar cheese; ½ cup cut up ham steak
+ ¼ cup salsa
+ 1 slice whole grain bread with 1 tablespoon low-sugar jelly
+ 1 cup low-salt V8 juice

Makes 1 serving. Per serving: 500 calories, 43 g protein, 42 g carbohydrates, 16 g fat (5 g saturated), 5 g fiber

BREAKFAST #4

+ 1 cup Greek yogurt with ½ cup strawberries or blackberries
+ ½ whole wheat bagel with almond butter
+ coffee or black tea

Makes 1 serving. Per serving: 327 calories, 17 g protein, 48 g carbohydrates, 7 g fat (3 g saturated), 6 g fiber

BREAKFAST #5

+ 1 cup whole grain fortified cereal with 1 cup 1% milk and topped with strawberries

+ 1 hard-boiled egg
+ green tea

Makes 1 serving. Per serving: 398 calories, 24 g protein, 60 g carbohydrates, 9 g fat (3 g saturated), 12 g fiber

---

BREAKFAST #6

+ 1 cup reduced-fat cottage cheese topped with cinnamon, 1 tablespoon chopped walnuts, and 1 sliced apple (with skin)
+ black tea

Makes 1 serving. Per serving: 332 calories, 32 g protein, 31 g carbohydrates, 10 g fat (3 g saturated), 6 g fiber

---

BREAKFAST #7

+ Breakfast Burrito (recipe on page 89) 1 whole egg and 2 egg whites; 2 tablespoons reduced-fat shredded Cheddar cheese, onions, peppers, salsa. Wrap in a whole-grain tortilla.
+ 1 orange
+ coffee or black tea

Makes 1 serving. Per serving: 285 calories, 22 g protein, 40 g carbohydrates, 7 g fat (3 g saturated), 5 g fiber

10 AM MID-MORNING SNACK

Your body needs 2 to 3 hours to break down the sugars in the food you ate for breakfast and convert them into energy. So around 10 or 10:30, it needs some more fuel. Go much longer than that without eating, and your energy will dip. What's more, you'll be so hungry for lunch, you're likely to head straight for the all-you-can-eat Chinese buffet.

Below are some good options for snacks. Team them with some lightly sweetened green or black tea. The sugar in it will boost your blood sugar, giving you some quick brain fuel, and the caffeine will improve your mental alertness. Tea counts toward your daily goal of 12 cups of water, and the compounds in the tea have been shown to boost metabolism. A Swiss study showed that men who drank green tea during the day burned more calories than men who drank water. USDA researchers got similar results in a study with black tea.

Eating protein- and fiber-rich meals or snacks every 3 hours helps keep your blood-sugar levels normal and your stomach from disturbing the 10 AM staff meeting. When it comes to blood sugar, you want homeostasis, not wild roller-coaster dips and jumps. Blood sugar ups and downs mess with your insulin resistance and can lead to prediabetes, elevated cholesterol, and high triglycerides. A snack at about this time also keeps your metabolic fire stoked, improving your body's ability to burn fat. Here are some easy, and tasty ideas for snacking.

SNACK #1
+ Deli-sliced turkey roll-ups

SNACK #2
+ 7 raw almonds
+ 1 stick string cheese

SNACK #3
+ Roll 1 slice deli turkey breast with 1 slice Swiss cheese

SNACK #4
+ Banana with 2 tablespoons almond butter or natural peanut butter

SNACK #5
+ 15 red grapes
+ ½ cup low-fat cottage cheese

SNACK #6
+ ¼ cup dry-roasted peanuts and walnuts mix
+ 1 cup low-fat (1%) chocolate milk

SNACK #7
+ ½ can Hormel Less Sodium Chili with Beans, microwaved

LUNCH

Lunch can be tricky, especially if you are eating out, because a lot of fast-food and cafeteria offerings are heavy on breads and pastas, which will crank up your blood sugar and make you feel sluggish after it dips. That's why brown-bagging your lunch will give you more control over what you eat. Aim for at least three servings of vegetables complemented with quality proteins, healthy

SMALL CHANGES, BIG RESULTS

Downsize your dinnerware with smaller bowls and plates. It works. Cornell researchers found that students scarfed down 59 percent more Chex Mix from large bowls than those who served themselves from small bowls.

fats, and complex carbs. Since vegetables are mainly water, fiber, and antioxidants, they will keep you hydrated and full with healthy calories.

Starting off with a spinach or spring-mix salad with colorful vegetables and a dressing of olive oil and vinegar is always good. Then get some protein by way of turkey, chicken, lean beef, cheese, fish, or beans. Here are some smart ideas using your list of **10 Foods to Eat Everyday.**

LUNCH #1
+ Tuna Sandwich
  Make with:
  2 slices 100% whole grain bread
  1 three-ounce can
  chunk light tuna in water, drained
  1 tablespoon light mayonnaise
  1 lettuce leaf
  2 slices tomato
  1 teaspoon chopped onions
  or celery
  2 dashes hot sauce

+ Medium apple with peanut butter
+ Water

Makes 1 serving. Per serving: 449 calories, 31 g protein, 61 g carbohydrates, 12 g fat (1 g saturated), 11 g fiber

LUNCH #2
+ Chef's Salad
  Make with:
  2 cups chopped romaine lettuce
  1 hard-boiled egg
  2 ounce piece, cubed
  turkey breast
  2 ounce pieced, cubed ham
  1 ounce sliced Swiss cheese
  or feta cheese
  6 cherry tomatoes
  olive oil and balsamic vinegar

Makes 1 serving. Per serving: 367 calories, 30 g protein, 12 g carbohydrates, 23 g fat (8 g saturated), 3 g fiber

LUNCH #3
+ Turkey/Avocado Wrap
  Make with:
  1 large whole wheat tortilla
  2 tablespoons hummus
  4 slices roast turkey breast
  2 slices red leaf lettuce or
  4 spinach leaves
  ¼ avocado, sliced

Makes 1 serving. Per serving: 310 calories, 29 g protein, 30 g carbohydrates, 12 g fat (2 g saturated), 8 g fiber

LUNCH #4

+ Peanut Butter and
  Sliced Apple Sandwich
  Make with:
  2 slices 100% whole grain and
  flaxseed bread
  2 tablespoons all-natural
  peanut butter or
  almond butter
  1 medium apple, cored
  and thinly sliced
+ 1 cup fat-free milk
+ 5 baby carrots with 2 tablespoons
  fat-free ranch dressing

Makes 1 serving. Per serving: 575 calories,
22 g protein, 86 g carbohydrates,
18 g fat (2 g saturated), 13 g fiber

LUNCH #5

+ 1 cup bean and beef chili
  with shredded Cheddar cheese
  and dollop of sour cream
+ 1 packet of whole-wheat crackers
+ 5 celery sticks
+ 1 apple
+ Unsweetened iced tea with lemon

Makes 1 serving. Per serving: 408 calories,
13 g protein, 63 g carbohydrates,
14 g fat (6 g saturated), 17 g fiber

LUNCH #6

+ 1 can sardines in water or olive oil
+ 6 whole grain crackers
+ 1 kosher pickle
+ 1 cup diet ginger ale or seltzer
+ 1 pear

Makes 1 serving. Per serving: 578 calories,
45 g protein, 44 g carbohydrates,
25 g fat (6 g saturated), 8 g fiber

LUNCH #7

+ Small garden salad with olive-oil
  and vinegar dressing
+ 1 slice cheese pizza

+ 1 orange
+ Water or seltzer

Makes 1 serving. Per serving: 675 calories,
24 g protein, 69 g carbohydrates,
35 g fat (2 g saturated), 9 g fiber

AFTERNOON SNACK

No time to break for a snack in the heat of a busy workday? You can't afford not to. In a study at the University of Massachusetts that analyzed the eating habits of 500 women and men, researchers found that people who ate a mid-afternoon snack to keep their metabolisms humming reduced their risk of becoming obese by 30 percent. Getting something good into your stomach between 3 and 4 PM may even improve your productivity by fueling your brain and boosting your attention and energy level. Plus, snacking at 4 PM will prevent feelings of sheer starvation at dinnertime.

SNACK #1

+ 4 halves deviled eggs
  made with hummus
  (mashed chickpeas)

SNACK #2
+ 1 cup Greek yogurt topped with ½ cup blackberries

SNACK #3
+ 1 inch square cheese block
+ 6 whole wheat crackers
+ 1 medium apple

SNACK #4
+ ¼ cup mixed nuts
+ 1 tangerine

SNACK #5
+ 1 apple, sliced, with 2 tablespoons natural peanut butter

SNACK #6
+ 10 baby carrots with 2 tablespoons reduced-fat ranch dressing
+ 1 cup calcium-enriched soy drink

SNACK #7
+ 1 Berry Roll-up (1 whole-wheat tortilla, 2 tablespoons low-fat cream cheese, ¾ cup mixed berries)

DINNER

Dinner for the 40+ man should be light in calories and heavy in nutrients. Eating too much at dinner can ignite your appetite and cause you to overeat late at night, setting you up for dangerous weight gain and uncontrollable hunger.

So, plan strategically. Begin with a vegetable soup, lentil or minestrone soup, or a low-calorie salad rich in high-fiber vegetables like broccoli, red cabbage, shredded carrots, sliced bell peppers, and dressed with olive oil and vinegar. Starting your meal this way will decrease your overall food consumption by up to 12 percent.

If you want to add a side starch to any of the entrees below, consider brown rice, which will add fiber to keep you full and kick down those late night cravings for pretzel rods. Use dinner to break the habit of cleaning your plate. Try to leave something starchy uneaten on your dinner plate.

DINNER #1
+ Grilled or Pan-fried Salmon with Broccoli and Beans
  Make with:
  1 five-ounce salmon fillet drizzled with olive oil and topped with cracked black pepper and lemon juice
  2 cups steamed broccoli
  ½ can red kidney beans
+ 1 cup mixed fresh berries with whipped cream for dessert

Makes 1 serving. Per serving: 675 calories, 52 g protein, 81 g carbohydrates, 18 g fat (5 g saturated), 26 g fiber

DINNER #2

+ Chicken Caesar Salad
  Make with:
  3 cups romaine lettuce
  1 grilled chicken breast
  ½ cup canned mandarin oranges
  2 tablespoons reduced-fat Caesar dressing
  1 tablespoon Parmesan cheese
+ 1 dark chocolate cookie with fat-free milk for dessert

Makes 1 serving. Per serving: 316 calories, 26 g protein, 43 g carbohydrates, 5 g fat (1 g saturated), 4 g fiber

DINNER #3

+ Steak with Brown Rice and Roasted Asparagus
  Make with:
  4 ounces filet mignon, grilled,
  1 cup cooked brown rice
  4 asparagus spears
+ Sugar-free lime Jell-O for dessert

Makes 1 serving. Per serving: 494 calories; 39 g protein; 48 g carbohydrate; 14 g fat (4 g saturated); 5 g fiber

DINNER #4

+ Spaghetti with Turkey Meatballs
  Make with:
  Whole grain spaghetti
  Mixture of ½ pound extra-lean ground round beef and ½ pound ground turkey breast
  Chopped onions, seasoned dry bread crumbs, 1 egg white, ¼ cup fat-free milk, two 28-ounce cans tomato sauce, one 15-ounce can diced tomatoes, 2 tablespoons Italian seasoning, 2 tablespoons sugar
+ ½ cup low-fat butterscotch pudding for dessert

Makes 6 servings. Per serving: 578 calories; 30 g protein; 99 g carbohydrates; 9 g fat; (3 g saturated); 12 g fiber.

DINNER #5

+ Chicken Fajitas
  Make with:
  Chicken breast strips with red bell peppers, onions, tomatoes, a teaspoon of olive oil and some chicken broth. Cook, stirring frequently.
  Whole wheat or soft corn tortillas
  Add sour cream, avocado slices, and salsa
+ ½ cup black beans.
+ 1 cup red grapes for dessert

Makes 1 serving. Per serving: 735 calories; 64 g protein; 71 g carbohydrate; 25 g fat (5 saturated); 10 g fiber.

DINNER #6

+ Grilled Tuna Steak with Cauliflower and Brown Rice
  Make with:
  1 tuna steak
  1 cup steamed cauliflower
  1 cup brown rice
+ ½ cup low-fat ice cream for dessert

Makes 1 serving. Per serving: 613 calories, 53 g protein, 68 g carbohydrates, 13 g fat (4 g saturated), 8 g fiber

DINNER #7

+ Turkey Meat Loaf with Steamed Spinach and Lentils
  Make with:
  ½ pound ground turkey breast
  ½ pound lean ground sirloin
  2 cups fresh spinach
  1 cup lentils, cooked
  Chopped onions, whole wheat bread crumbs, 2 eggs, ½ cup barbecue sauce
  + Chunk (1 oz.) of dark chocolate

Makes 4 servings. Per serving: 535 calories; 39 g protein; 59 g carbohydrates; 16 g fat (8 g saturated); 9 g fiber.

chapter 3

POWER FOODS FOR LIFE

40+ Delicious Ways to Lose Weight, Get Fit, and Look Fantastic

RACK INTO A PLATE of steaming, fragrant Alaskan king crab legs, or swallow a delicious zinc supplement followed by a strontium chaser. Here's another: a fresh-from-the-sea shimmering Blue Point oyster or a spoonful of Geritol. Are you getting the picture?

Let's face it: Eating real food is a lot more fun than gobbling supplements. And all the key nutrients that you need to stay healthy in your 40s and beyond—zinc, calcium, copper, boron, potassium, magnesium, folic acid, lutein, beta-carotene, selenium, sulforaphane, phosphorus, lycopene, and dozens and dozens of beneficial vitamins, flavonoids, and polyphenols— are right there in fresh, whole, natural foods.

Besides, most supplements simply can't compare to the real thing. Consider the findings of the Iowa Women's Health Study. This large investigation of 34,492 women found that those who ate foods rich in vitamin E lessened their chances of ➡

suffering a stroke, but women who took vitamin E supplements were not protected.

Natural foods contain thousands of compounds that interact in complex ways, and if you take one out, there's no predicting how it will function on its own, according to Frank Hu, MD, PhD, professor of nutrition and epidemiology at the Harvard School of Public Health. That's not to say that taking a multivitamin isn't worthwhile "health insurance," but large-scale trials of individual antioxidant supplements have been largely disappointing.

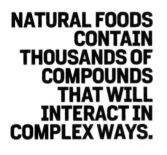

NATURAL FOODS CONTAIN THOUSANDS OF COMPOUNDS THAT WILL INTERACT IN COMPLEX WAYS.

You can get most, if not all, of the nutrients essential to health by selecting the right combination of foods. But you have to know where to look. The last chapter offered a minimalist approach to healthy eating, based on a simple diet with just 10 core foods to amp up your weight-loss efforts while maintaining good nutrition. Here, we're going to expand your repertoire of nutritional superfoods with many more options that specifically address the dietary needs of the 40+ body. These are the best foods for healthy hearts, bones, muscles, brains—even better sex. Build these foods into your diet monthly, if not weekly. If you notice a duplicate or two from Chapter 2, that's because some of these foods are powerful enough to belong on both lists. Eat them twice as much. Later on, we'll show you how to make some delicious meals from these good things.

MUSCLE MAKERS:
WHERE TO FIND THE PROTEIN

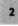

CHOCOLATE MILK

Low-fat chocolate milk is a terrific postexercise recovery drink because it contains whey protein, which helps muscles recover and repair. In addition, it delivers both calcium and vitamin D, which research shows are important for preserving cartilage and joint health. A 2006 study in the *International Journal of Sport Nutrition and Exercise Metabolism* found that low-fat chocolate milk is as good as or better than Gatorade for replacing glucose in fatigued muscles.

2

GRASS-FED BEEF

Most of the beef in your local supermarket comes from grain-fed cattle; that's a major source of the omega-6 fatty acids that make it into our bodies. Not to be confused with the heart-healthy omega-3 fatty acids you get from oily fish, omega-6s have been shown to contribute to inflammation, which causes all kinds of bodily havoc over time. The fatty acids in grass-fed beef, by contrast, contain more of the omega-3 variety. Grass-fed beef also contains conjugated linoleic acid (CLA), which studies have shown helps to reduce belly fat and build lean muscle. Two servings of lean grass-fed beef— flank or tenderloin, for example—a week is a good amount to shoot for.

QUINOA

This nutty-tasting grain has fewer carbohydrates than regular cereal grains, some healthy fats, and— get this—about twice the protein. In fact, it's considered a "complete" protein, like eggs, because it contains all of the essential amino acids your body needs for muscle growth. Try to get quinoa into your weekly meal plan, using it as a substitute for brown rice or sweet potatoes. You'll find it in the rice aisle or health food section of your supermarket. Quinoa can be used to make pilafs, risottos, salads, and soups, even as breakfast cereal with a sprinkling of cinnamon.
➡ **TRY THIS EASY QUINOA SALAD RECIPE.** *Boil 1 cup quinoa in a mixture of 1 cup pear juice and 1 cup water. Let cool. In a large bowl, toss 2 diced apples, 1 cup fresh blueberries, ½ cup chopped walnuts, and 1 cup plain fat-free yogurt.*

4

NONFAT RICOTTA

Made from whey, this soft cheese is rich in amino acids, which speed muscle recovery after a workout. Flavor it with jam and spread it on a cracker. Use it as you would cottage cheese. Top a whole wheat pizza crust with it. Or put half a cup in a blender with skim milk and fruit for a postworkout cheesecake-flavored smoothie— and a good source of protein and calcium.

HOW I EAT

"I eat four meals a day, and each one is based on a different type of protein. Breakfast comes from the dairy or egg group—four egg whites plus one yolk is one of my favorites. Lunch is trail mix: a half-cup mixture of walnuts, peanuts, raisins, and cranberries. I eat two dinners! The first is at 5:30, before I exercise, and includes fish with beet relish and corn salsa. Around 8:30, I eat a poultry-based dinner. It's the perfect post-workout meal because it floods my muscles with amino acids and minerals—everything they need for repair and recovery."

— **MICHAEL DANSINGER, MD, AGE 41,** *Obesity researcher at Tufts–New England Medical Center in Boston*

5

LENTILS

Lentils provide protein, B vitamins, and zinc, which is important for good sexual health. Eat half a cup twice a week. Put them in soups, add them to stews, and even sneak them into lasagna. They are dried so you have to cook them for about 30 minutes. Or soak them for an hour in cold water, then cook them for 15 minutes.

6

EGGS

Don't worry. You can eat a couple a day without getting into cholesterol trouble. Recent studies have shown that the fat in the yolk is important to keep you satiated, and the benefits of the minerals and nutrients in the yolk outweigh its cholesterol effect. Calorie for calorie, eggs deliver more biologically usable protein than any other food, including beef. In addition, eggs contain vitamin B12, which is necessary for fat breakdown and muscle contraction, plus folate, vitamins D and E, selenium, phosphorus, iron, and zinc. Eggs from chickens fed omega-3–laced feed will provide you with 100 milligrams of those fats per egg—another way to get the important fatty acids without eating more fish.

7

TOFU

To get a full complement of amino acids as well as isoflavones, which help muscles recover from exercise, try pressed soybean curds—known and loved by nutritionists as tofu. Tofu is the great food chameleon; it has no real flavor, which means you can dump it into any dish and it will take on the flavor of the sauce or dressing while bulking up the meal with healthy plant protein. Marinate it for stir-fries, and toss it into salads and soups.

Best Food Sources of Resveratrol

Resveratrol, a flavonoid found in grape skins, grape juice, and wine, has been shown to protect arteries, lower LDL cholesterol, and help fight cancer by inhibiting cell growth. Here's where to find it.

+ Blueberries
+ Dark chocolate
+ Grapes
+ Lingonberries

+ Peanuts
+ Peanut butter
+ Pistachios

+ Pomegranate juice
+ Red wine
+ Red grape juice

+ Unsweetened cranberry juice
+ White grape juice
+ White wine

BONE BUILDERS:

FOR A STRONG STRUCTURE

8

ALASKAN KING CRAB

High in protein and low in fat, the sweet flesh of the king crab is spiked with zinc—a whopping 7 milligrams per 3.5-ounce serving. "Zinc is an antioxidant, but more important, it helps support healthy bone mass and immune function," says Susan Bowerman, RD, assistant director of the Center for Human Nutrition at the University of California at Los Angeles. "Several studies have linked adequate zinc intake to increased immunity and decreased incidences of respiratory infection." And you can reap all these benefits by swapping one of your weekly fish meals for a 6-ounce serving of crab.

9

KIWIFRUIT

Like bananas, this fuzzy fruit is high in bone-protecting potassium. Freeze them for a refreshing energy kick, but don't peel the skin: It's edible and packed with nutrients such as vitamin C.

10

OYSTERS

Shellfish, in general, are an excellent source of zinc, calcium, copper, iodine, iron, potassium, and selenium. It's best not to eat shellfish too often, as they contain some mercury, but don't pass them up when you get the chance. Two

The Perfect Plate

How to envision a leaner you every time you sit down to eat

Keep this simple diagram in mind to ensure the correct portions of the three main food categories. High-fiber fruits and vegetables should take up one half of the plate. One third of the plate is reserved for meat, fish, or vegetable protein, and a bit less than ¼ of the remaining space can be for your starch. Eating this way will train you to naturally serve yourself more low-calorie vegetables and still eat satiating protein and some fat at every meal.

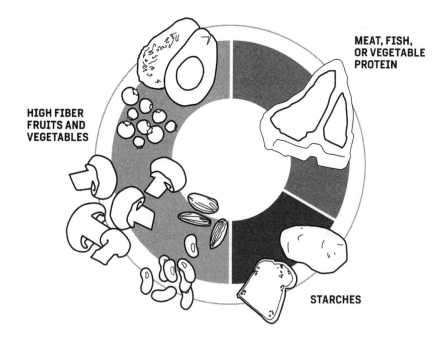

MEAT, FISH, OR VEGETABLE PROTEIN

HIGH FIBER FRUITS AND VEGETABLES

STARCHES

servings of shellfish (12 ounces) a week are safe, according to the U.S. Food and Drug Administration and Environmental Protection Agency.

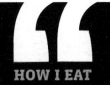

11

PRUNES

These tasty dried plums are rich in copper and boron, both of which can help prevent osteoporosis. The fiber in them, inulin, creates an acidic environment in the gut when broken down by intestinal bacteria, which, in turn, improves calcium absorption.

12

BOK CHOY

This crunchy cruciferous vegetable is more than the filler that goes with shrimp in brown sauce. Bok choy is rich in bone-building calcium, as well as vitamins A and C, folic acid, iron, beta-carotene, and potassium. Potassium keeps your muscles and nerves in check while lowering your blood pressure.

BANANAS

Long known for their ability to ease high blood pressure, bananas are rich in potassium, an electrolyte that also helps prevent the loss of calcium from the body. Bananas bolster the nervous system, boost immune function, and help the body metabolize protein. One banana packs a day's worth of potassium, and its carbohydrate content speeds recovery after strenuous exercise.

14

LEEKS

These scallionlike cousins of garlic and onions are packed with bone-bolstering thiamine, riboflavin, calcium, and potassium. Leeks are also rich in folic acid, a B vitamin that studies have shown lowers levels of the artery-damaging amino acid homocysteine in the blood.

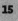

ARTICHOKES

This fiber-rich plant contains more

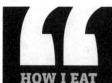

HOW I EAT

I try to minimize carbohydrate intake, including complex carbohydrates, and replace some of the calories with protein and fat. Last night for dinner, I had 80 percent lean ground beef, browned, and stuffed inside green bell peppers that were cored out. We baked them and added some shredded Cheddar cheese."

— **JEFF VOLEK, PhD, RD, AGE 40** *Nutrition and exercise researcher at the University of Connecticut at Storrs, and associate editor of the journal* Nutrition and Metabolism

bone-building magnesium and potassium than any other vegetable. Its leaves are rich in flavonoids and polyphenols—anti-oxidants that can cut the risk of stroke—and vitamin C, which helps maintain the immune system.

16

SPINACH

Spinach builds muscle, increases bone-mineral density (thus protecting against osteoporosis), and reduces fracture rates. It's also rich in calcium, phosphorus, potassium, zinc, and even selenium, which may help protect the liver and ward off Alzheimer's disease. One more reason to add it to your diet: A study in the *Journal of Nutrition* suggests that the carotenoid neoxanthin in spinach can kill prostate cancer cells, while the beta-carotene fights colon cancer.

17

BROCCOLI

Easy to find, broccoli is loaded with the potent nutrient sulforaphane, which studies at Johns Hopkins University suggest has powerful anticancer properties. Other good sources of this phytonutrient include cauliflower, kale, Brussels sprouts, and cabbage.

IMMUNITY BOOSTERS:

FOODS THAT FIGHT DISEASE

18

GREEN TEA

Studies show that green tea—infused with the antioxidant EGCG—reduces the risk of most types of cancer. The phytonutrients in tea also support the growth of intestinal bacteria and inhibit the growth of dangerous E. coli, Clostridium, and Salmonella.

19

CINNAMON

Fragrant, spicy cinnamon is rich in antioxidants that inhibit blood clotting and bacterial growth. Studies also suggest that it may help stabilize blood sugar,

Your Rainbow Coalition against Aging

Mix up a palate of colorful vegetables on your plate to boost antioxidant power

To fully benefit from these disease-fighting compounds, you need to combine them with a little fat. For example, Ohio State University researchers found that people who ate a salad topped with half an avocado absorbed 5 to 10 times more beta-carotene and lutein—carotenoids found in carrots and spinach, respectively—than those who had salads without the fatty avocado. And eating avocado with salsa boosted the absorption of lycopene—a carotenoid in tomatoes—by almost five times. Drizzling some heart-healthy olive oil over your vegetables or dipping raw vegetables into full-fat ranch dressing or a bit of melted cheese would have the same effect.

GREEN	YELLOW & ORANGE	RED	BLUE & PURPLE	WHITE
Spinach, collard greens, and broccoli are rich in lutein, which keeps your vision sharp.	Carrots, pumpkin, corn, sweet potatoes, and melon contain carotenoids, which reduce the risk of developing cancer and cataracts.	Tomatoes and watermelon are loaded with lycopene, which may protect your body against cancer and heart disease.	Blueberries and blackberries contain anthocyanins, powerful anti-inflammatories that also suppress the growth of tumors.	Garlic, onions, and cauliflower contain sulfur compounds that may ward off some cancers.

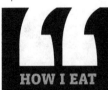

HOW I EAT

I make breakfast easy so it's hard to miss. It's a bowl of yogurt mixed with Grape Nuts cereal and topped with almonds and berries every day. It's important to have protein at every meal because it's satiating. Whole grain cereals are high in fiber, and that's important for gastrointestinal function—and it makes you more full and tides you over. Plus, your body uses more calories to break down high-fiber foods. The yogurt provides protein and a little fat. People worry about fat, but this extra protein and extra fat also contribute to that feeling of being full. The other important thing I try to do is get more food earlier in the day and eat less at dinner. The key to doing that is to put something in your stomach in the late afternoon, some celery with peanut butter, maybe, so you're not starving at dinnertime. And start the dinner meal with a salad or a vegetable soup to provide the fill-factor."

— LESLIE BONCI, RD, MPH, AGE 52
Registered dietitian, director of nutrition, UPMC Center for Sports Medicine, nutrition consultant for the Pittsburgh Steelers, author of Sport Nutrition for Coaches.

reducing the risk of type 2 diabetes. And it may also reduce LDL cholesterol.

20

CHILI PEPPERS
Chilis are powerful medicine, able to stimulate the metabolism, thin the blood, and help release endorphins, natural pain- and stress-reducing brain chemicals. Chilis are also rich in beta-carotene, which turns into vitamin A in the blood and fights infections, as well as capsaicin, which inhibits chemicals that cause inflammation.

21

GINGER
If you have motion sickness, chewing on a bit of ginger will help quell the queasiness. Chop ginger or grind it fresh, and add it to soy marinades for fish, chicken, or tofu. One of the special nutrients in ginger is gingerol, a cancer suppressor that studies have shown to be particularly effective against cancer of the colon.

22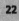

SWEET POTATOES
Go sweet instead of white for health benefits. Sweet

potatoes contain glutathione, an anti-oxidant that can enhance nutrient metabolism and immune–system health, as well as protect against Alzheimer's, Parkinson's, liver disease, cystic fibrosis, HIV, cancer, heart attack, and stroke—and prevent diabetes.

23

BLUEBERRIES

They contain more antioxidants than any other fruit. Buy them fresh or frozen out of season. They're not just a topping for breakfast cereals and ice cream. Grab a handful to munch on in the afternoon.

24

FIGS

Packed with potassium, manganese, and antioxidants, this fruit also helps support proper pH levels in the body, making it more difficult for pathogens to invade. Plus, the fiber in figs can lower insulin and blood–sugar levels, reducing the risk of metabolic syndrome.

25

TOMATOES

Tomatoes are rich in heart-healthy lycopene, which also helps protect against degenerative brain disease and cancer. Cooked tomatoes and tomato paste deliver the most lycopene, so even your slice of pizza can be considered a health food. Just don't overdo the cheese.

26

MUSHROOMS (REIKI, SHIITAKE, MAITAKE)

Toss them in salads, of course, or sauté with red wine, which contains the antioxidant resveratrol and magnifies their immunity-boosting power. Mushrooms are rich in the antioxidant ergothioneine, which protects cells from abnormal growth.

27

POMEGRANATES

This trendy fruit contains some of the planet's most powerful cancer-fighting polyphenols and ellagitannins, which give the fruit its color.

INFLAMMATION FIGHTERS:

BEATING THE ENEMY OF LONG LIFE

28

BING CHERRIES

Research by the U.S. Department of Agriculture shows that eating up to 45 bing cherries a day can lower the risk of tendonitis, bursitis, arthritis, and gout. Studies also suggest that cherries reduce the risk of chronic diseases and metabolic syndrome. Even richer in anti–inflammatory compounds are tart cherries and cherry juice, says nutritionist Leslie Bonci, RD, of the UPMC Center for Sports Medicine. "Toss dried tart cherries into yogurt or salads, or make a smoothie with tart cherry concentrate," she suggests.

29

TURMERIC

Spice up grilled or broiled fish and chicken with turmeric and get the benefit of a polyphenol called curcumin, which has cancer-fighting and anti-inflammatory properties. Studies show that it also inhibits the growth of plaque associated with Alzheimer's disease.

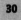

PINEAPPLE

This sweet, juicy fruit packs a potent mix of vitamins, antioxidants, and enzymes that reduce inflammation and protect against colon cancer, arthritis, and macular degeneration.

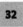

APPLES

Apples are packed with inflammation-fighting antioxidants, one of the most powerful being quercetin. Studies show that eating apples may cut stroke and heart disease risk by 25 percent and diabetes by 27 percent.

32

OLIVE OIL

Extra-virgin olive oil is rich in beneficial monounsaturated fats and polyphenols that reduce inflammation in cells and joints. A study in the journal *Nature* found that it's as effective as Advil at reducing inflammation.

33

WILD FATTY FISH

Go wild or go home. Mackerel, sardines, salmon, and other and other wild fatty fish contain a hearty dose of omega-3 fatty acids, which protect the heart, cells, joints, and brain. The DHA and EPA in the oil of these fish also reduce the risk of colorectal cancer. Farmed fish contain too much omega-6 fatty acids from the feed they are given.

34

FLAXSEED

Rich in protein and fiber, these nutty-tasting seeds are great on cereal and yogurt. The oil in them is high in alpha-linolenic acid, the plant-based omega-3 fat that makes flaxseed, like fish, a terrific food for both brain and heart.

ALMONDS

An ideal afternoon snack, these nuts are rich in fiber and plant sterols, which lower bad cholesterol. They're also rich in amino acids, which support muscle growth.

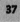

DARK CHOCOLATE

The flavonoids in dark chocolate inhibit platelet clumping, which reduces the risk for stroke, heart attack, and embolism. It's high in calories, so limit yourself each day to half a bar with at least 70 percent cacao.

37

WHOLE GRAINS

Get the whole package with whole grains such as oatmeal, wheat berries, wild rice, quinoa, barley, and brown rice. Whole grains are high in fiber and calm inflamed tissue while keeping the heart strong and the colon healthy. Be sure to read nutrition labels and look for "100 percent whole grain flour." "Whole wheat flour" is still refined, a process that breaks down the grain and strips it of its nutrients.

LIBIDO LIFTERS:
FOODS FOR BETTER SEX

38

POMEGRANATE JUICE
A study in *The Journal of Urology* found that pomegranate juice may reduce the risk of sexual dysfunction.

39

GRILLED SHRIMP SALAD
Not to be confused with chopped up shrimp in a mayonnaise bath; look for a green salad and add grilled shrimp. The little swimmers are full of zinc—good for your little swimmers—and leafy greens are full of folate. Both can boost sperm levels.

40

OATMEAL
Oats produce a chemical that releases testosterone into the blood supply, increasing sex drive and orgasm strength.

Mix in some honey for an added boost.

41

SWISS CHARD
Swiss chard is a potent source of magnesium, which helps dilate blood vessels, say Japanese researchers.

42

HONEY
Honey's B vitamins aid the production of testosterone, and its boron content helps the body use estrogen, which is key for proper bloodflow and arousal.

43

BLACKBERRIES
The soluble fiber in blackberries ushers cholesterol through your digestive tract before it chokes your arteries. The berries also contain compounds that improve circulation for a natural Viagra–like effect.

chapter 4

HOME-COOKED FAT BURNERS

Great-tasting Recipes
Using the Best Power Foods
for Fitness at 40+

EFF ALEXANDER IS spreading himself thin, and he's starting to feel fat.

Just 2 years ago, the 43-year-old folded his business and took a job at a major international computer company. It's a rewarding position, he says, but the work is wreaking havoc on his body. "My butt is beginning to take the shape of my desk chair," he complains. Meanwhile, he's either working late or entertaining clients so often that more than half his meals come with a bill at the end of them.

"I feel like I'm holding everything together on the business end, but in this economy, there never seems to be a break. What free time I do have is dedicated to playing with my 2-year-old or stealing away for a catnap." And the strain is beginning to show, especially around Alexander's waistband.

His dilemma is the classic catch-22: The older a man gets, the higher he rises in his career, but the harder it is for him to ➡

manage his food supply. Success today means traveling by car, train, or plane; making deals over lunch at the Steak and Gristle; and working the rubber-chicken circuit.

But finding time to eat at home more often—to control what goes into your body so you can get more out of it—is the key to looking and feeling healthier. It may help to earn a paycheck that's healthier as well. Indeed, being overweight also makes it harder to climb the corporate ladder. Overweight men are considerably more likely than their normal-weight peers to be passed over for a promotion. Surveys show that they also earn an average of $4,000 less each year.

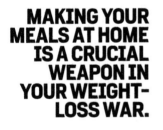

MAKING YOUR MEALS AT HOME IS A CRUCIAL WEAPON IN YOUR WEIGHT-LOSS WAR.

So no matter how stressed you might feel, good, healthy food is worth the effort, as we will show you. And making your meals at home is a crucial weapon in your weight-loss war. You'll learn how to choose healthy ingredients with the most nutrition per calorie, and you can control portions—the key to weight-loss success!

The good news is that good food doesn't necessarily have to take long to prepare. On the following pages, we've compiled more than 20 healthful breakfasts, lunches, and dinners using many of the 40+ nutritional powerhouse ingredients listed in chapter 3. Many of these meals take less than 15 minutes to prepare; some involve just one pot, so there'll be very little cleanup. Best of all, these meals offer varied tastes and textures. Sample one or two of these recipes, and you won't be so eager to run out to a restaurant. You'll find there's better eating right at home.

BREAKFAST BURRITOS WITH VEGETARIAN SAUSAGE

- 2 large egg whites, lightly beaten
- 4 vegetarian sausage links
- 4 whole wheat tortillas (10" diameter)
- 2 scallions, thinly sliced
- 1 large, ripe avocado, pitted, peeled, and sliced
- 1 medium-size tomato, diced
- ¼ cup sour cream

Coat a small nonstick skillet with cooking spray. Heat over medium-high heat. Pour in the egg whites. Cook, stirring occasionally, for 3 to 4 minutes or until the egg whites are the consistency you like.

While cooking the eggs, microwave the sausage links for about 1 minute 30 seconds. Cut into bite-size pieces.

Divide the egg whites into four quarters with a spatula. Put a quarter of the egg onto each tortilla. Top with some of the sausage, scallion, avocado, tomato, and sour cream, and roll up.

Makes 4 servings. Per serving: 397 calories, 14 g protein, 46 g carbohydrates, 17 g fat, 4 g sat fat, 7 g fiber, 660 mg sodium

BREAKFAST OATMEAL AND NUTS

- ½ cup steel-cut oats
- 1 cup water or 2% milk
- ¼ cup chopped walnuts
- 1 tablespoon maple syrup

Combine the oats and water or milk in a medium saucepan over medium-high heat. Bring to a boil. (Use more or less liquid to reach desired consistency.)

Reduce heat. Cook gently, just below the boiling point, for 5 minutes or until the mixture is the consistancy you like.

Top with the walnuts and maple syrup.

Makes 1 serving. Per serving: 440 calories, 11 g protein, 51 g carbohydrates, 23 g fat, 2 g sat fat, 7 g fiber, 4 mg sodium

➡ **QUICK BITE:** Walnuts are loaded with vitamin E, an antioxidant that bolsters the immune system. Steel-cut oats are whole oats that have been chopped into smaller pieces. This oatmeal is denser, creamier, and chewier and delivers the most fiber. Rolled oats are steamed, rolled, and flaked for quicker cooking. They are better for you than "instant" oats, which are essentially powdered oats that produce a bowl of paste (and are often loaded with sugar).
Go for the steel-cut or rolled oats to get the most nutrition.
Instead of topping with maple syrup, shave some dark chocolate over the hot oatmeal for a hit of flavor and added antioxidants.

SPEEDY EGG BURRITO

2 omega-3 eggs
1 cup frozen mixed vegetables
  (black beans, peppers, corn)
1 whole wheat tortilla
  (10" diameter)
½ cup low-fat shredded
  Cheddar cheese
¼ cup salsa

Beat the eggs in a medium bowl. Stir in the mixed vegetables. Spread the mixture on a microwaveable plate coated with nonstick spray.

Microwave for 1 minute. Stir with a fork, and microwave again until the eggs are cooked.

Spoon into the tortilla. Top with shredded cheese and salsa. Fold, and roll.

Makes 1 serving. Per serving: 468 calories, 33 g protein, 38 g carbohydrates, 23 g fat, 11g sat fat, 5 g fiber, 1089 mg sodium

➡ *QUICK BITE:* The ideal breakfast should pack at least 20 grams of protein and 5 grams of fiber to give your body a high-quality, long-lasting, steady supply of energy. This meal does it in less than 5 minutes. Omega-3 eggs come from hens given feed rich in omega-3 fatty acids.

THREE-EGG VEGETABLE OMELET

2 tablespoons chopped onions
2 tablespoons chopped
  green bell peppers
2 tablespoons sliced fresh
  mushrooms
¼ cup broccoli florets
2 egg whites + 1 large whole
  omega-3 egg, well beaten

Coat a large, nonstick skillet with olive oil cooking spray, and heat over medium heat.

Add the onions, peppers, mushrooms, and broccoli. Cook, stirring frequently until soft. Transfer to a bowl. Set aside.

Coat the skillet with spray again. Add the eggs, allowing them to cover the bottom of the pan.

Cook for 3 minutes, or until the bottom begins to set.

Top one half of the omelet with the vegetable mixture. Carefully fold the remaining half over the filling. Cook the eggs until they are cooked through.

Makes 1 serving. Per serving: 152 calories, 17 g protein, 10 g carbohydrates, 4 g fat, 1 g sat fat, 3 g fiber, 200 mg sodium

Flash Breakfasts

When you don't have time to cook, you still have time to slap together a nutritious morning meal. These 9 breakfasts come together superfast

1

½ cup cottage cheese topped with blueberries, strawberries, or raspberries

2

Kashi GoLean high-protein, high-fiber cereal with fat-free milk

3

1 scoop whey protein powder mixed in vanilla-flavored organic low-fat milk

4

1 slice sprouted grain bread with 1 tablespoon natural peanut or almond butter

5

1 whole wheat tortilla with one slice each of turkey and cheese

6

2 slices roast beef rolled in a slice of Swiss or white American cheese

7

½ cup Greek yogurt topped with strawberries and chopped walnuts

8

2 microwaveable vegetable-protein sausages on a hotdog roll or a slice of whole wheat bread, topped with organic low-sugar ketchup

9

½ cup vanilla yogurt topped with a handful of All-Bran Extra Fiber cereal and blueberries

GREEN EGGS AND HAM CUPS

1   pkg frozen chopped spinach
3   eggs
½   cup shredded reduced-fat Cheddar cheese
¼   cup finely chopped green bell peppers
¼   cup finely chopped onions
¼   cup chopped ham steak

Preheat the oven to 350ºF. Spray a 12-cup muffin pan with nonstick cooking spray.

Cook the spinach in the microwave or on the stove top according to package directions. Drain well.

Whisk the eggs in a medium bowl. Stir in the spinach, cheese, peppers, onions, and ham. Mix well.

Dividing the mixture evenly, fill each muffin cup. Bake for 20 minutes, or until an inserted toothpick comes out clean. The recipe makes enough for a small crowd. Or you can refrigerate the leftovers for several quick breakfasts.

Makes 6 servings. Per serving: 75 calories, 8 g protein, 3 g carbohydrates, 3 g fat, 1 g sat fat, 1 g fiber, 229 mg sodium

EGG MCMOUNTY MUFFIN

1   egg + 1 egg white
1   slice Canadian bacon
1   whole wheat English muffin
1   slice American cheese
1   tablespoon pure maple syrup

Coat a small nonstick skillet with cooking spray. Heat the skillet over medium heat. While the skillet is heating, beat the eggs in a small bowl. When the skillet is hot, pour in the eggs.

Let the eggs cook undisturbed over medium heat until they begin to get hard. Gently stir them off the bottom and move them to the side. Place the bacon in the skillet.

Toast the English muffin.

When the eggs are cooked to the consistency you like and the bacon slice is warmed, place them on one half of the muffin. Top with the slice of cheese. For a little sweetness, drizzle the teaspoon of maple syrup (more to taste) onto the top muffin half.

Makes 1 serving. Per serving: 414 calories, 27 g protein, 44 g carbohydrates, 14 g fat, 6 g sat fat, 4 g fiber, 1178 mg sodium

TURKEY AND HUMMUS WRAP

1 whole wheat tortilla
  (10" diameter)
2 tablespoons hummus
  (mashed chickpeas)
¼ cup roasted red pepper strips
4 slices roast turkey breast
4 or 5 spinach leaves or 2 large
  romaine lettuce leaves

Lay the tortilla flat on a large cutting board. Spread the hummus evenly over the tortilla to within ½ inch of the edge. Lay the peppers evenly over the hummus. Layer the turkey and the spinach or lettuce.

Fold in the sides and roll to form a wrap. Cut diagonally in half.

Makes 2 servings (½ wrap each).
Per serving: 241 calories, 36 g protein,
18 g carbohydrates, 4 g fat, 0 g sat fat,
2 g fiber, 620 mg sodium

SPICY MANHATTAN CLAM CHOWDER

2 slices bacon
2 ribs celery, thinly sliced
1 onion, finely chopped
1 clove garlic, minced
2 6½-ounce cans chopped clams
¾ cup bottled clam juice
1 large potato, peeled and cubed
2 carrots, chopped
1 teaspoon dried thyme
1 bay leaf
1 14-ounce can diced tomatoes
  Hot-pepper sauce to taste

Cook the bacon in a large saucepan over medium heat until crisp. Transfer to a plate lined with paper towels. Crumble into a small bowl. Set aside.

Add the celery, onion, and garlic to the bacon drippings in the saucepan. Cook, stirring occasionally, or until the onion and celery are tender.

Drain the juice from the clams into a small bowl. Set the clams aside. Add the juice to the onion mixture. Stir in the bottled clam juice, potato, carrots, thyme, and bay leaf. Bring to a boil. Reduce the heat to low. Cover and simmer for 20 minutes.

Stir in the tomatoes with their juice. Bring to a boil over high heat. Reduce the heat to low. Add the reserved clams. Cover and simmer for 8 minutes. Discard the bay leaf. Season with the hot–pepper sauce. Stir in the bacon.

Makes 4 servings. Per serving: 231 calories,
28 g protein, 20 g carbohydrates,
3 g fat, 1 g sat fat, 5 g fiber, 556 mg sodium

CHICKEN AND GRAPES SALAD SANDWICH

1	pound boneless, skinless chicken breast
½	cup low-fat plain Greek yogurt
3	tablespoons low-fat mayonnaise
1	tablespoon Dijon mustard
¼	teaspoon garlic powder
½	teaspoon salt
¼	teaspoon ground black pepper
¼	cup finely chopped onion
½	cup finely chopped celery
½	cup seedless red grapes, sliced in half
6	Lettuce leaves
12	slices whole grain bread

Put the chicken breasts in a medium saucepan and cover with water. Bring to a boil over high heat, then reduce to low and cook gently, just below the boiling point, for about 10 minutes, or until the meat is no longer pink inside. Remove the chicken from the pan and allow to cool on a cutting board. Cut into small cubes.

Place the yogurt, mayonnaise, mustard, garlic powder, salt, pepper, onion, and celery in a large bowl. Mix well.

Fold the chicken chunks into the mixture, then add the cut-up grapes and mix gently.

Place ½ cup of the chicken mixture and a lettuce leaf between two slices of whole grain bread to make one serving.

Makes 6 servings (1 sandwich each).
Per serving: 258 calories, 23 g protein,
34 g carbohydrates, 6 g fat, 1 g sat fat,
10 g fiber, 836 mg sodium

➡ *QUICK BITE:* **The next time you cook chicken, cook some extra breasts to have on hand for chicken salad. Cutting the traditional mayonnaise with the yogurt dials back the fat grams and calories.**

SPEEDY FISH TACOS

1 tablespoon canola oil
1 clove garlic, minced
½ teaspoon dried oregano
¼ teaspoon ground cumin
2 6-ounce cans chunk
white tuna packed in water,
drained and flaked
1 14-ounce can diced
tomatoes with zesty jalapeños,
well drained
¼ teaspoon hot-pepper sauce
Juice of ½ a lime
4 8" whole wheat tortillas
1 cup shredded low-fat
Monterey jack cheese

Mix the oil, garlic, oregano, and
cumin in a 1–quart microwaveable
dish. Microwave 60 seconds,
or until heated through.

Stir in the tuna, tomatoes, hot
sauce, and lime juice.

Microwave for 2 to 4 minutes, or
until heated through, stopping once to
stir. Warm the tortillas by microwaving
them for 5 to 10 seconds.

Spoon some of the hot filling
into each tortilla, top with cheese,
and fold up.

*Makes 4 servings. Per serving: 306 calories,
32 g protein, 25 g carbohydrates,
10 g fat, 4 g sat fat, 3 g fiber, 896 mg sodium*

➡ **QUICK BITE:** This meal takes just
5 minutes to prepare and 6 to cook.

HOMEMADE GUACAMOLE

2 medium-size ripe avocados,
pitted and peeled
½ cup seeded and chopped
tomatoes
¼ cup finely chopped red onion
¼ cup finely chopped fresh cilantro
2 tablespoons lime juice
2 teaspoons seeded and minced
jalapeño peppers
¼ teaspoon sea salt
Pinch of ground cumin

Mash the avocado with a large
fork or potato masher in a medium
bowl. Use a wooden spoon to mix
in the tomatoes, onion, cilantro,
lime juice, jalapeños, salt, and cumin.
Serve immediately or cover and chill
in the refrigerator.

*Makes four ½–cup servings.
Per serving: 172 calories, 2 g protein,
11 g carbohydrates, 15 g fat, 2 g sat fat, 7 g fiber,
154 mg sodium*

➡ **QUICK BITE:** Use a spoonful of
guacamole instead of mayonnaise
on your next sandwich. The heart-
healthy monounsaturated fat in the
avocado will keep you feeling full
longer, and it will improve absorption
of vitamins A, D, E, and K from the
sandwich and other foods you eat.

THE RECIPES
DINNER

LINGUINE WITH VEGETABLES

1½ cups cooked whole wheat
linguine
1 clove garlic, minced
2 teaspoons olive oil
1 cup broccoli florets
1 cup sliced yellow squash
1 cup cut asparagus spears
Salt and freshly ground pepper

Cook the linguine according to
package directions.

Heat 1 teaspoon of he oil in a large
saucepan over medium–high heat.
add the garlic and cook, stirring
frequently until lightly brown.

Add the broccoli, squash, and
asparagus, and stir frequently
until slightly soft.

Add the cooked pasta and remaining
olive oil. Mix the pasta and vegetables
well to distribute the oil and heat the
pasta. Season with salt and pepper.

*Makes 1 serving. Per serving: 444 calories,
19 g protein, 73 g carbohydrates,
12 g fat, 2 g sat fat, 16 g fiber, 223 mg sodium*

➡ ***QUICK BITE:*** Whole–wheat pasta
is better for you than the kind made
with processed white flour. We like
Barilla PLUS multigrain pastas.

SESAME TOFU WITH BOK CHOY AND CORN

2 tablespoons sesame seeds
1 16-ounce package firm
tofu, drained and cut into
bite-size cubes
4 teaspoons toasted sesame oil
1½ pounds baby bok choy,
cut into 1" pieces
2 tablespoons finely chopped
fresh ginger
3 cloves garlic, minced
1 15-ounce can baby corn, drained
and rinsed

Place the sesame seeds in a medium
bowl. Add the tofu cubes and gently
roll them around to coat.

Heat 2 teaspoons of the oil in a
medium nonstick skillet over medium
heat. Add the tofu and cook, turning
occasionally, until golden brown on all
sides, about 10 minutes. Transfer tofu
to a plate lined with paper towels.

Heat the remaining oil in a wok or
large nonstick skillet over high heat.
Add the bok choy, ginger, and garlic,
and cook, stirring constantly for
4 minutes, or until soft. Add the baby
corn and continue cooking and
stirring for 2 minutes longer.
Toss in the tofu and heat through.

*Makes 4 serving. Per serving: 297 calories,
18 g protein, 31 g carbohydrates,
15 g fat, 2 g sat fat, 5 g fiber, 135 mg sodium*

➡ ***QUICK BITE:*** To drain tofu,
place between two plates lined with
paper towels and let stand for
30 minutes so the towels can absorb
the excess liquid.

PROSCIUTTO-WRAPPED HALIBUT WITH ASPARAGUS

12	large spears asparagus, ends trimmed off
½	tablespoon extra-virgin olive oil
2	tablespoons chopped parsley
½	tablespoon lemon juice
4	halibut fillets
4	thin slices prosciutto ham
2	teaspoons canola oil
½	teaspoon ground black pepper

Preheat the oven to 350°F.

Boil a large pot of water. Fill a large bowl halfway with cold water and a half-dozen ice cubes.

Cook the asparagus in the boiling water until cooked through but not soft, 7 to 8 minutes. Remove using long tongs and place them in the ice water bath to stop the cooking. Once cooled, remove and pat dry with paper towels.

Make a vinaigrette by mixing the olive oil, parsley, and lemon juice in a small bowl.

Sprinkle the halibut fillets with the pepper and wrap each with a slice of the prosciutto.

Pour the canola oil in a large nonstick ovenproof skillet and heat it over medium-high heat on the stove top.

Cook the ham-wrapped fish, seam side down, for about 2 minutes, then flip over to the other side, until the prosciutto is crisp on both sides. Turn the fish over to seam side down, then transfer the pan to the oven and bake until the fish flakes easily, or about 4 minutes (depending on the thickness of the fillets).

Place a fillet on a dinner plate with three asparagus spears, and top the asparagus with a spoonful of the vinaigrette.

Makes 4 servings. Per serving: 209 calories, 29 g protein, 3 g carbohydrates, 8 g fat, 1 g sat fat, 1 g fiber, 437 mg sodium

OVEN-ROASTED MISO SALMON

- 3 tablespoons white miso
- 1 tablespoon mirin (a rice-based wine similar to sake but with a lower alcohol content)
- ³/₈ teaspoon low-sodium soy sauce
- 1 teaspoon canola oil
- 4 6-ounce wild-caught salmon fillets
- 1 teaspoon sesame seeds, toasted
- 1 scallion, green part only, thinly sliced

Preheat the oven to 400°F.

Whisk the miso, mirin, and soy sauce in a bowl until blended. Set aside.

Add the oil to a large nonstick ovenproof skillet on the stove top over medium–high heat. Add the salmon, skin side up, and cook for 2 to 3 minutes, or until lightly browned.

Flip the fish over and place the skillet in the heated oven. Roast until the salmon is opaque, or about 6 to 8 minutes.

Brush the salmon with the miso mixture. Sprinkle with the sesame seeds and garnish with the scallion.

Makes 4 servings. Per serving: 296 calories, 35 g protein, 7 g carbohydrates, 13 g fat, 2 g sat fat, 1 g fiber, 466 mg sodium

➡ **QUICK BITE:** A recent study linked Japanese men's high fish consumption with raised levels of omega–3 fatty acids and a lower incidence of heart disease.

SPICY SEAFOOD STEW

- 1 tablespoon olive oil
- ½ cup chopped onions
- ½ cup chopped red bell peppers
- 1 clove garlic, minced
- 1 28-ounce can diced tomatoes with juice
- 1 28-ounce can tomato sauce
- ¼ cup dry red wine
- ¼ cup chopped fresh parsley
- 1 teaspoon Worcestershire sauce
- ¼ teaspoon crushed red peppers
- 8 ounces bay scallops
- 8 ounces medium shrimp, peeled and deveined
- 1 10-ounce can whole baby clams

Spread olive oil over the bottom of a large stock pot and heat over medium–high heat.

When the oil is hot, add the onions, bell peppers, and garlic. Cook, stirring frequently, for 5 minutes, or until the onion is tender.

Dump in the undrained tomatoes, tomato sauce, wine, oregano, parsley, Worcestershire sauce, and red peppers. Stir well. Bring to a boil over medium heat, then reduce the heat to simmer. Cover and cook gently, just below the boiling point, stirring occasionally, for 20 minutes.

Add the scallops, shrimp, and clams. Bring to a boil over medium heat, then reduce the heat to simmer. Stir. Continue cooking gently, stirring often, for 8 minutes or until the scallops are tender and the shrimp turn pink.

Ladle into soup bowls.

Makes 6 servings. Per serving: 288 calories, 37 g protein, 22 g carbohydrates, 5 g fat, 1 g sat fat, 4 g fiber, 1380 mg sodium

GINGERED BEEF WITH BROCCOLINI AND WALNUTS

2 tablespoons oyster sauce

2 tablespoons finely chopped fresh ginger

1 tablespoon low-sodium soy sauce

1 teaspoon chili paste with garlic

5 tablespoons water

2½ teaspoons toasted sesame oil

1½ pounds broccolini, trimmed and cut into bite-sized pieces

¾ pound lean flank steak, cut across the grain, into thin strips (no thicker than ½")

6 scallions, trimmed and cut into 1" pieces

⅓ cup chopped walnuts, toasted

Whisk together the oyster sauce, ginger, soy sauce, chile paste, and 2 tablespoons of the water in a small bowl. Set aside.

Heat the oil in a wok or large nonstick skillet over high heat. Add the broccolini, and cook, stirring constantly, for 3 minutes, or until soft. Add the remaining water and continue cooking and stirring for 2 minutes.

Add the steak, scallions, and the oyster sauce mixture and continue cooking and stirring for 1 minute, or until the beef is just cooked through. Stir in the walnuts and serve.

Makes 4 servings. Per serving: 280 calories, 25 g protein, 15 g carbohydrates, 15 g fat, 3 g sat fat, 5 g fiber, 714 mg sodium

➡ *QUICK BITE:* Broccolini, often called "baby broccoli," is a sweet, tender hybrid of broccoli and Chinese chard. This delicate vegetable contains high amounts of vitamin C, potassium, fiber, and vitamin A. It's delicious brushed with olive oil and grilled, then topped with a sprinkle of coarse sea salt and lemon juice.

WHITE BEAN AND CHICKEN CHILI

1 tablespoon olive oil

2 onions, chopped

2 cloves garlic, minced

3 pounds boneless,
skinless chicken breasts,
cut into bite-size pieces

2 14-ounce cans fat-free,
reduced-sodium chicken broth

4 15.5-ounce cans cannellini beans,
drained and rinsed

1 4.5-ounce can chopped green
chile peppers with juice

1 teaspoon salt

1 teaspoon ground cumin

¾ teaspoon dried oregano

½ teaspoon chili powder

½ teaspoon ground black pepper

⅛ teaspoon ground cloves

⅛ teaspoon ground red pepper

Heat the oil in a large pot over medium–high heat. Add the onions, garlic, and chicken. Cook, stirring frequently, for 6 minutes, or until the chicken is lightly browned.

Transfer the contents of the pot to a 4–quart pot or large slow cooker. Add the broth, beans, undrained chile peppers salt, cumin, oregano, chile powder, black pepper, cloves, and red pepper. Stir well.

Cook on low heat for 4 hours. Uncover and cook for 1 more hour, stirring occasionally.

Makes 6 servings. Per serving: 488 calories, 64 g protein, 37 g carbohydrates, 8 g fat, 1 g sat fat, 11 g fiber, 929 mg sodium

➡ **QUICK BITE:** This meal is perfect for the slow cooker because it takes just 10 minutes to prepare. Put the cooker on low and it will cook all day and be ready for dinner (or it can be ready in as little as 5 hours). The cannellini beans are rich in magnesium, iron, and folate. Rinsing them will wash away some of the added sodium. Try them in salads or add them to soups for a fiber and protein boost.

CHICKEN MARSALA

3 tablespoons whole wheat flour
¼ teaspoon white flour
¼ teaspoon ground white pepper
1½ pounds chicken cutlets, or chicken breast meat, pounded thin
2 cups sliced mushrooms
2 tablespoons thinly sliced shallots
1 cup Marsala wine
½ cup low-sodium chicken broth
2 tablespoons chopped parsley
½ teaspoon chopped fresh thyme leaf

Combine flours and pepper in a shallow bowl. Dredge the chicken in the mixture and set aside.

Lightly coat a large nonstick skillet with cooking spray and heat on medium–high. Add the chicken to the skillet and sauté until lightly browned, 2 to 3 minutes per side. Remove the cutlets to a plate and keep them warm.

Add the mushrooms and shallots to the skillet. Stir for 1 to 2 minutes.

Add the wine to the skillet. Boil to evaporate moisture, scraping any loose brown bits from the bottom of the skillet.

Reduce heat and add the broth, parsley, and thyme. Stir. Cook just at the boiling point, stirring frequently until the volume of the broth mixture reduces by half.

Return the chicken to the skillet and cook gently, just below the boiling point, for 5 minutes, or until the cutlets are heated through.

Makes 4 servings. Per serving: 325 calories, 42 g protein, 15 g carbohydrates, 3 g fat, 1 g sat fat, 1 g fiber, 495 mg sodium

➡ **QUICK BITE:** Serve with side dishes of mashed red potatoes and boiled glazed carrots, a combo that adds only 113 calories per serving. Mash ½ cup of boiled red potatoes with the skins left on for added fiber and nutrients. Mix in 1 tablespoon of fat-free cream cheese, 1 tablespoon of fat-free milk, and salt and pepper to taste. After boiling ½ cup of peeled, sliced carrots, drain them and stir in 1 tablespoon of honey to glaze them.

chapter 5

LOOSEN UP TO STAY FIT

A Flexible Body Makes Everything Feel Better

F YOU HATE TO STRETCH BEFORE A WORKOUT, you're in good company. Most men would rather avoid it, and those who say they like it are probably lying. Stretching is boring and burns too much time in our heavily scheduled lives. Even athletes would rather skip it if they could. It's a lot more fun to pump some iron and build muscles to flex than to stretch the old hamstrings.

But flexibility is so important to good health, especially as you enter your 40s, when joints begin to lose some motion and lubrication. That's the decade when, typically, musculoskeletal imbalances become progressively worse, causing pain and compromising mobility, says Harold Millman, DPT, a doctor of physical therapy in private practice in Bethlehem, Pennsylvania.

Sure, you want to be limber enough to reach down for a quarter on the street without throwing out your back, but more crucial to the 40+ body is avoiding the damaging postural imbalances that come with tight muscles and a sedentary lifestyle. ➡

"Our daily dominant position is—what? It's sitting," says Millman. "We sit at work, we sit in the car, at the computer when we get home." And that hunched-over-the-keyboard posture in your 40s and 50s creates imbalances that over time may develop into a rounded-shoulder, slump-backed "old-lady slouch" that's more typical of people in their 60s and 70s.

STRETCHING WILL GET TO THE ROOT OF MOST MUSCULAR PAIN AND IMBALANCE ISSUES.

"Compounding the problem of too much sitting is the fact that our pectorals (chest muscles) are so much larger and stronger than our trapezius and rhomboids (back muscles) and pull everything forward, so you keep getting that rounded look," Millman says. Belly fat adds to this imbalance and can create chronic muscular pain and tension. What can you do? Try our stretching program, which will get to the root of most muscular pain issues that aren't triggered by athletic overuse in the 40-year-old desk jockey.

+EASY STRETCHES TO DO AT WORK
WAKE UP, REJUVENATE, AND BE MUCH MORE PRODUCTIVE

TIGHTNESS IN THE SHOULDERS, NECK, AND BACK often leads to fatigue, injury, soreness, and lack of mobility. It's a casualty of the modern desk job. Good flexibility allows a muscle to lengthen and the joints to operate through a full range of motion. When muscles are elastic, your posture improves and you breathe deeper. Using more lung capacity sends more oxygen-rich blood to your brain to keep you alert and productive.

Employ the 20-20 rules, advises Alan Hedge, PhD, a professor of ergonomics at Cornell University. Every 20 minutes, stand for 20 seconds and stretch or shake things out. "Just 20 seconds away from your computer screen reduces fatigue and increases blood circulation," says Hedge. Now you'll have the power to sit up straight.

Every 2 hours at work, try the following series of postural correction moves and rejuvenating stretches that will make tight muscles feel great and improve your oxygen efficiency.

THE DRILL	DURATION
Chest Elevation	10 seconds/5–10 reps
Scapular Retraction	10 seconds/5–10 reps
Chin Tuck	10 seconds/5–10 reps
Upper Cervical Spine Flex	10 seconds/5–10 reps
Upper Back and Neck Strengthening	10 seconds/5–10 reps
Rhomboid Range of Motion	10 seconds/5–10 reps
Corner Chest Stretch	15 seconds/5–10 reps

CHEST ELEVATION

Sit in a chair with your arms at your sides and your feet flat on the floor. Gently raise your chest toward the ceiling, but don't look up. Keep your chin level with the floor.

➡ **Hold this position for 10 seconds, then relax, and repeat 5 to 10 times.**

SCAPULAR RETRACTION

Get into the position for the **CHEST ELEVATION** stretch while sitting, but this time place your hands on your hips. Squeeze your shoulder blades together, feeling the stretch in your chest.

➡ **Hold for 10 seconds, then relax, and repeat the sequence 5 to 10 times.**

CHIN TUCK

Assume the **CHEST ELEVATION** position while sitting. Keeping your chin level with the floor, pull your chin, head, and neck inward (not down).

➡ **Hold for 10 seconds, then relax and repeat.**

TIP: **Placing your finger on your upper lip may help guide your head through the proper range of motion and correct any mistakes.**

UPPER CERVICAL SPINE FLEX

From the **CHEST ELEVATION** position while seated, dip your head forward slightly as if you were nodding "yes." Feel the stretch in the neck at the base of the head.

➡ **Pause for 10 seconds, then relax and repeat 5 to 10 times.**

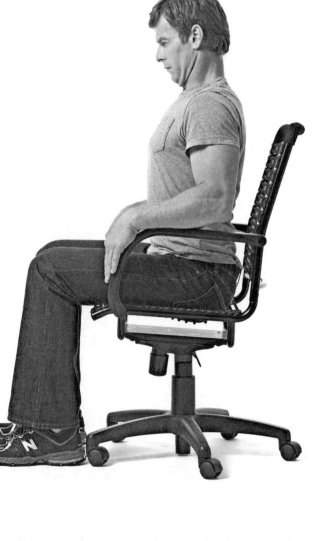

DYNAMIC LUMBAR STABILIZATION

This is less of a stretch and more of an exercise in teaching your body to recognize the neutral position of the spine, which is the safest position for lifting, working, and playing sports like golf and tennis.

When your torso is in the neutral position, you get the least joint compression and vertebral stress and the strongest muscular corset. In other words, learning to stand this way will save you a lot of trouble down the road.

To find the position, stand straight and contract your abdominal muscles. Tilt your pelvis forward and backward until you find the position of optimum balance.

➡ **TIP: Do this daily to correct postural imbal-ances due to having a large belly or top-heavy chest.**

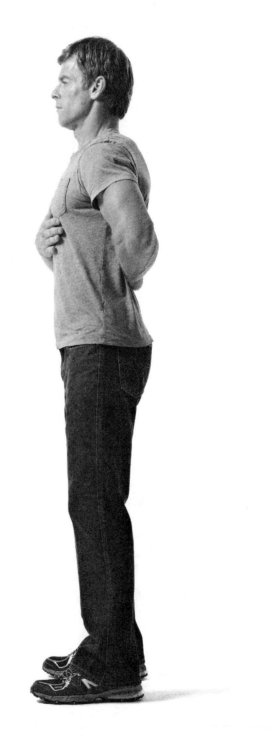

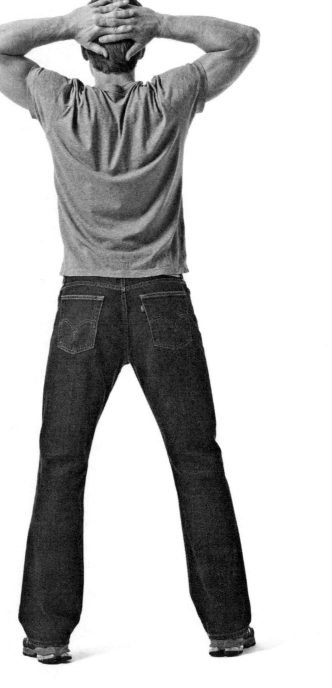

UPPER BACK AND NECK SCAPULAR STRENGTHENING

To strengthen the rhomboids, try this version of the scapular retraction.

Stand upright. Clasp your hands behind your head. Flex your elbows back while pinching your shoulder blades together.

➡ **Hold for 10 seconds, then relax, and repeat 5 to 10 times.**

**RHOMBOID
RANGE
OF MOTION**
Stand upright. Clasp
your hands behind you
at the small of your back.
Pinch your shoulder
blades together.
➡ **Hold for 10 seconds,
then relax, and repeat
5 to 10 times.**

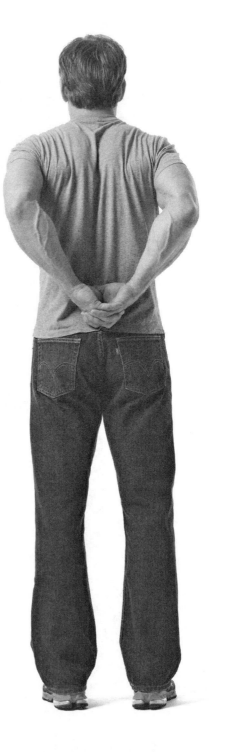

CORNER CHEST STRETCH

Stand facing the corner of a room. Raise your hands to shoulder height, and place your forearms, elbows, and hands against each wall. Lean inward to stretch your chest muscles.

➡ **Hold for 15 seconds or until you feel loose.**

TIP: By raising or lowering the position of your arms, you can alter the stretch to focus on different parts of the pectorals.

+EASY STRETCHES TO DO AT HOME
A FLEX ROUTINE FOR MORNING, NIGHT, OR WHILE WATCHING TV

THE REST OF THESE STRETCHES are a bit more difficult to do at work, so save them for home. They are great to do in the morning to lengthen your muscles after sleeping all night. But move around a bit first to get the blood flowing to your limbs before attempting to stretch. You can do these in the morning, at night, or any time you're feeling tight.

THE DRILL	DURATION
Lower Back Extension	5 seconds/5-10 reps
Back Stretch Sequence	See page 118
Shoulder and Arms Stretch Sequence	5 seconds/5-10 reps
Hamstring Stretch	30 seconds per leg
Quadriceps Stretch	30 seconds per leg
Rotational Hip Flexor Stretch	15 seconds/5-10 reps per leg

BACK AND SHOULDERS

LOWER BACK EXTENSION

Lie on the floor on your stomach. Place your hands slightly in front of your shoulders. Keeping your hips down and using only your arm muscles, push your upper body up as far as you can before it becomes painful.
➡ **Hold for 5 seconds, then relax, and repeat 5 to 10 times.**

BACK STRETCH SEQUENCE

1 Get on your knees and place your hands in front of you on the seat of a chair or an exercise ball. Sit back on your heels and contract your abdomen to increase the stretch in your lower back.

➡ **Hold for 5 seconds,** relax, and repeat 5 to 10 times

2 Place your hands shoulder-width apart on the floor and face the ground. Now gently arch your back toward the ceiling while tucking your butt in.

➡ **Hold for 5 seconds, relax, and repeat 5 times.**

3 After your last arch, immediately lower your butt until it touches your heels. Allow your arms to stretch out in front of you and let your back relax in a straight, neutral position (no arch in either direction).

➡ **Hold for 30 seconds.**

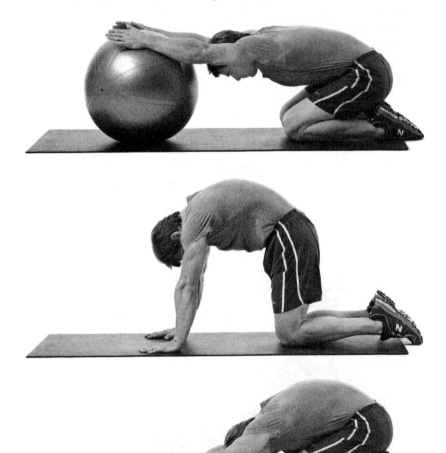

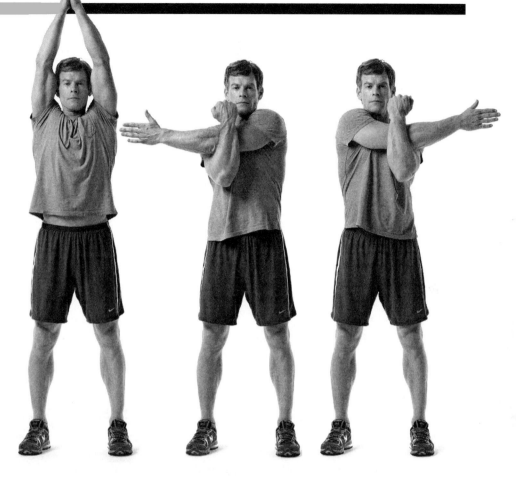

SHOULDER AND ARMS STRETCH SEQUENCE

The rotator cuff is made up of four small muscles that cover the shoulder joint and keep your arm centered in place while you do your daily reaching, pushing, yanking, and Frisbee tossing. Stretching the shoulder joint keeps it flexible and helps with stability. Do these three moves to *keep it healthy.*

1 Raise both arms overhead and place your palms together. Concentrate on standing as tall as possible and reaching as high as you can.

➡ **Hold the stretch for 5 seconds, then repeat 5 to 10 times.**

2 This is called the anterior shoulder stretch. Stand straight with your legs comfortably spaced. Raise your left arm to shoulder height and move it across your body, keeping it parallel with the floor. Now hold your left upper arm with your right arm and pull forward until you feel the stretch in the back of your shoulder. Be sure to keep the left upper arm against your chest throughout the move.

➡ **Hold for 5 seconds, relax, and repeat 5 to 10 times. Repeat the exercise with your right arm.** ➡

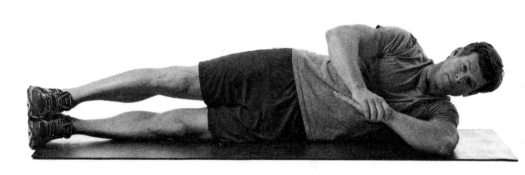

SHOULDER AND ARMS STRETCH SEQUENCE (CONTINUED)

3 Lie on the floor on your left side. Bring your left arm out to the side so that your forearm and upper arm form a right angle at the elbow.

Stabilize your shoulder against the floor. Now, keeping your upper arm on the floor, press your forearm back toward the floor with your right hand.

➡ **Hold for 5 seconds, rest, and repeat 5 to 10 times.**

Next, push your left forearm upward with your right hand as far as it will go before becoming painful.

➡ **Hold for 5 seconds, rest, and repeat 5 to 10 times. Switch to your right side and repeat the sequence with your right arm.**

HIPS AND LEGS

HAMSTRING STRETCH

This lengthens the hamstrings and the lower back muscles. Lie down and bend your right knee to 90 degrees to stabilize your hips, and press the small of your back against the floor. Keeping your left knee as straight as possible, lift that leg off the floor with your hands clasped behind your knee. (It may help to hook the middle of a towel over your foot's arch and hold the ends in your hands to increase the stretch). While pulling your leg vertically, you'll feel the stretch in the back of your thigh.

➡ Hold this position for 30 seconds. Then repeat with the right knee straight. *TIP:* You will find that you can get a deeper stretch if you press your outstretched leg forward for a few seconds while holding your leg back with your hands or the towel. Relax, then gently try to pull your leg in farther.

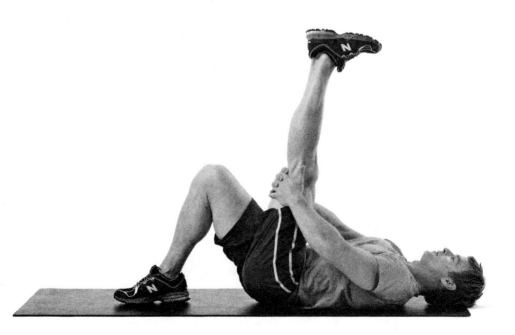

QUADRICEPS STRETCH

Your quads are the four big muscles in the front of the legs. They help you flex your hips and extend your legs, and they are responsible for keeping your kneecaps centered on your legs. Important muscles, your quads— so stretch them daily. Here's how:

Stand with your feet together and your hips straight. This is important. A common mistake is putting the hips forward and creating an arch in the back when you start to bend your knee and raise a foot. Got it right?

Okay, now bend your left knee back so you can grab your left foot over the laces of your running shoes. Pull your foot back toward your butt and make sure that your thigh remains vertical. Remain standing in the neutral position.

➡ **Hold the stretch for 30 seconds, before repeating the stretch with your right leg. _TIP:_ If you have trouble balancing, try focusing your gaze on a point in front of you.**

ROTATIONAL HIP FLEXOR STRETCH

Place your left foot on a bench with your knee bent at 90 degrees. Keeping your back leg straight and toes pointing forward, lean forward until you feel the stretch in the hip and the back of the leg.

➡ **Hold for 5 seconds. Now shift your pelvis from side to side, 5 times, holding each position for 5 seconds. Release and repeat the stretch sequence with your right foot on the bench and your left leg back.**

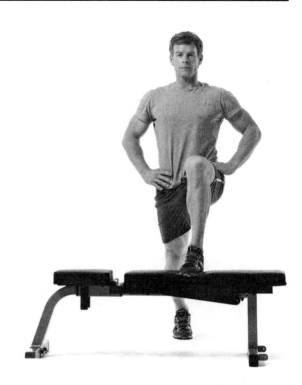

123

+THE FOAM ROLLER STRETCHES
GIVE YOUR MUSCLES A MASSAGE

A HIGH-DENSITY FOAM ROLLER is a terrific stretching tool for the 40+ body because it combines self-massage, bringing warming blood to the muscle tissue, while you elongate your muscles. Made of closed cell foam, these rollers come in a variety of shapes and sizes. We recommend the versatile 36-inch round model shown here, which can be ordered from Power-Systems.com and other suppliers for about $20.

THE DRILL	DURATION
IT band stretch	10–30 seconds/5–10 reps
Upper-Back	10–30 seconds/5–10 reps
Quadriceps Stretch	10–30 seconds/5–10 reps
Hamstring Stretch	10–30 seconds/5–10 reps
Butt Stretch	10–30 seconds/5–10 reps

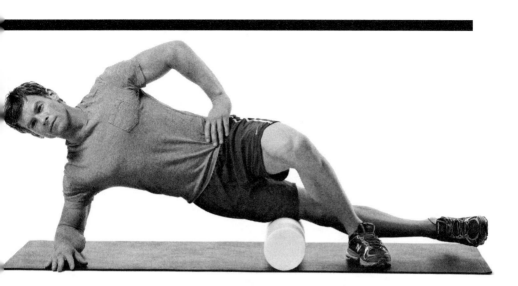

IT BAND STRETCH

Your illiotibial band runs from your knee to your hip and can often become tight, especially for runners. To stretch it out: Assume a side plank position, then slip the foam roller between the knee and hip. If you are lying on your right side, as shown, bring your left leg over your right for support. Slowly roll back and forth until you find the pressure point, then stretch there for 10 to 30 seconds. Release, then roll and find the spot again.

➡ **Repeat several times. Then turn over and stretch the IT band of your left leg.**

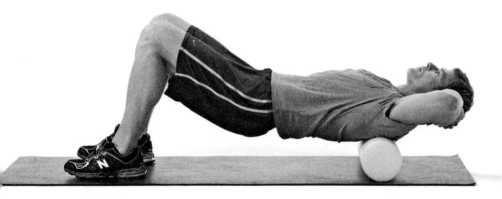

UPPER-BACK STRETCH

Place a foam roller under your upper back, near your shoulderblades. With your feet flat on the floor and your hands behind your head, stretch your back over the roller. You can roll back and forth slightly to massage the muscle, but don't roll near your lower back or risk injury. Try this option: Position the foam roller lengthwise so that it supports your entire spine, and roll from side to side for a full-back massage.

QUADRICEPS STRETCH

From a pushup or plank position, slip a foam roller under your thighs. Holding your body straight and contracting your abs, roll yourself back and forth over the roller.

➡ **Stretch for 10 to 30 seconds and repeat 5 to 10 times.**

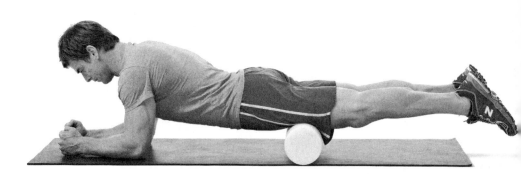

HAMSTRING STRETCH

Sit on a foam roller with your legs outstretched, and support yourself with your arms behind you. Postion yourself so the roller is directly under your hamstrings. Slowly roll forward and back from your butt to the bend in your knee.

➡ **Stretch for 10 to 30 seconds and repeat 5 to 10 times.**

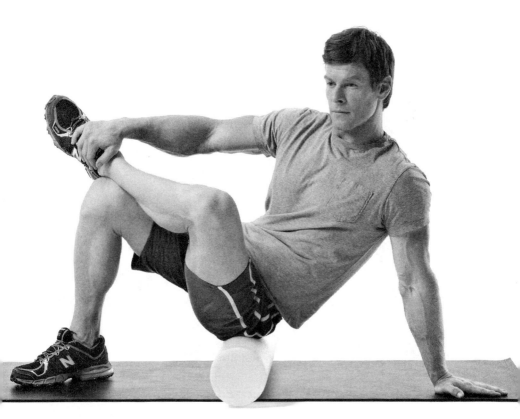

BUTT STRETCH

The piriformis is the butt muscle through which your sciatic nerve runs. When inflamed or tight, it can trigger numbing low-back pain. This stretch/massage will work wonders. Sit on a foam roller and support yourself with one arm. Now, lift one leg and place it across the other bent knee. One butt cheek should be on the roller, the other lifted off. Roll until you find the painful hot spot.

⇒ Hold that position for 10 to 30 seconds, rolling to massage the piriformis. Relax and repeat 5 to 10 times before switching positions and performing the stretch on the other side of the glutes.

+STRETCHING BEFORE EXERCISE

A WARMUP BEFORE A WORKOUT IS CRUCIAL FOR THE 40+ BODY

LACK OF FLEXIBILITY IS A HUGE PROBLEM for people who are attempting to get back in shape, because they often exercise without first priming their muscles for the stress of all that running, jumping, and twisting. It's sort of like trying to run your car without lubrication; the engine will seize up without oil. By the same token, if you don't get blood flowing to your muscles, your body won't move as well and you'll risk tearing something or developing imbalances. And you'll pay a lot more to an orthopedic surgeon than you would to an auto mechanic!

Stretching prepares your muscles, joints, and connective

tissues for your workout. It elevates your core temperature and improves blood flow to your tissues, lengthens and loosens tight muscles and ligaments, and, when performed correctly, can even strengthen and stabilize the body's critical core of abdominal, lower back, and gluteal muscles that are engaged in nearly every movement you make.

"One of the biggest mistakes people make is not stretching in three planes of motion," says Ron DeAngelo, director of sports performance training at the UPMC for Sports Medicine in Pittsburgh. "You need to stretch in all the directions your body moves to get the real benefit of the exercise."

ONE OF THE BIGGEST MISTAKES PEOPLE MAKE IS NOT STRETCHING IN THREE PLANES OF MOTION.

The three planes of movement DeAngelo refers to include the frontal plane (side to side motion), the sagital plane (frontward to backward motion), and the transverse plane (rotational motion). When you run, you may think you're only moving in the sagittal plane but you're actually doing all three. By stretching in all three planes, you make your body able to move as it was biomechanically meant to move. When tight muscles restrict, this normal movement can lead to muscle pulls or joint injuries.

"Your body will always favor the path of least resistance, even if it's the wrong way to move. Flexibility removes those obstacles," says DeAngelo.

On the following pages, you'll find some terrific dynamic and static stretches. Depending upon your sport of choice, you may want to add a stretch that mimics a specific repetitive move. But this group will warm up your entire body for whatever you have in mind. Do this stretching routine to warm up before every workout. The calf stretch, hamstring stretch, quad stretch, butt stretch, and anterior shoulder stretch make up a good cooldown after a workout to flush lactic acid from your muscles. Or choose your own favorite cooldown stretches. Also, try to stretch a bit on your day(s) off from exercise.

Stretching for Exercise
Here's how to warm-up and cool down when working out

WARMUP STRETCHES	DURATION
Prisoner Squat	10–15 reps
Trunk Rotation	10 reps
Knee Hug to Lunge	10 reps with each leg
Inch worm	5 reps
Hip Circle	10 reps with each leg
Hamstring stretch	30 seconds with each leg
Butt stretch	30 seconds with each leg
Airplane	5 reps with each leg, hold 10 seconds
Back Lunge and Twist	10 reps with each leg
Butterfly stretch	15–30 seconds
Calf stretch	30 seconds
Anterior shoulder stretch	15 seconds with each arm

COOLDOWN STRETCHES	DURATION
Calf stretch	30 seconds
Hamstring stretch	30 seconds with each leg
Butt stretch	30 seconds with each leg
Quad stretch	30 seconds with each leg
Anterior shoulder stretch	15 seconds with each arm

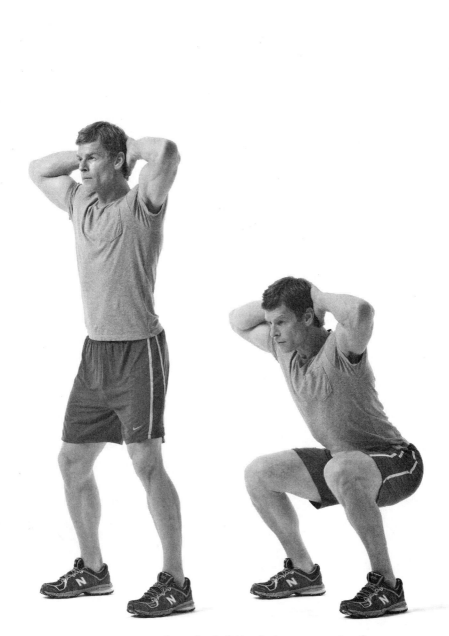

PRISONER SQUAT

Stand with your hands behind your head, your chest out, and your elbows back. Sit back at your hips and bend your knees to lower your body as far as you can without losing the natural arch of your spine. Squeeze your gluteals and push yourself back to the starting position.

➡ **Do 10 to 15 reps.**

TRUNK ROTATION
Stand with feet shoulder–
width apart and hands on
your hips. Keeping your
back straight, bend
forward at the hips. Then
begin leaning to the right,
then rotating around the
back, then to your left,
and back to the forward
position in a smooth,
circular motion. Avoid
jerky stops at each
position. You should
keep your hips stable
and make circles with
your upper body.
➡ **Do five starting to
the right and then five
starting to the left.**

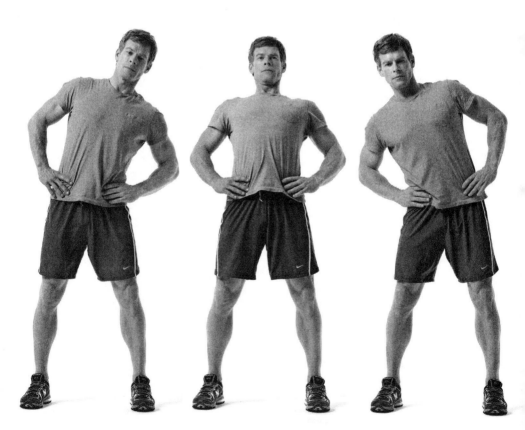

KNEE HUG TO LUNGE

Stand with your feet together. Hug your left knee to your chest. Let go of the knee and step into a lunge. *(Be sure to keep your knee aligned above your ankle—never more forward—to avoid injury.)* Step back, lifting your knee again.

➡ **Do 10 reps, then repeat the lunge with your right leg.**

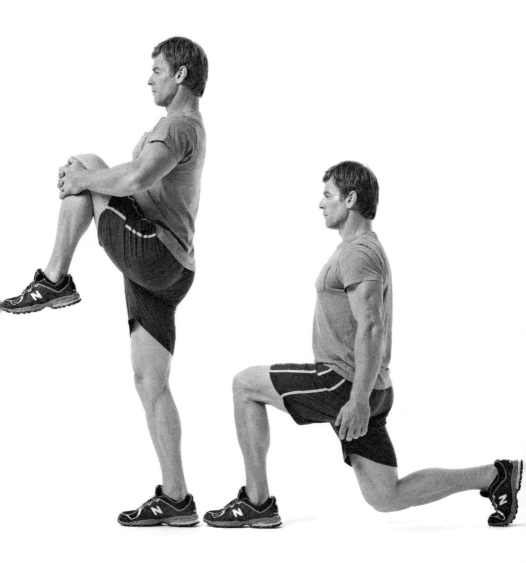

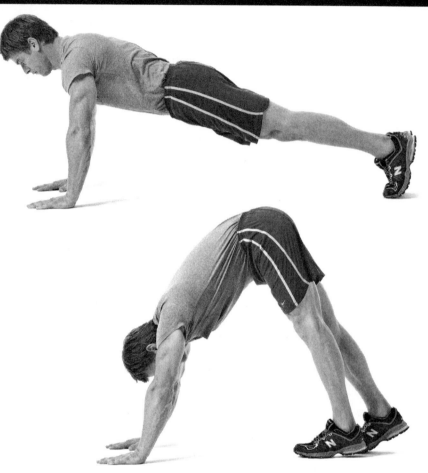

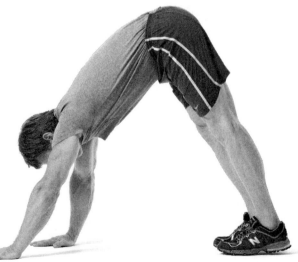

INCH WORM

Start in a pushup
position. Slowly walk your
feet toward your hands.
Your heels can come off
the floor, but stop walking
forward when the stretch
in the backs of your
legs starts to feel
uncomfortable. Keeping
your feet still, slowly walk
your arms forward until
you are back in the
pushup position.

➡ **Perform 5 times.**

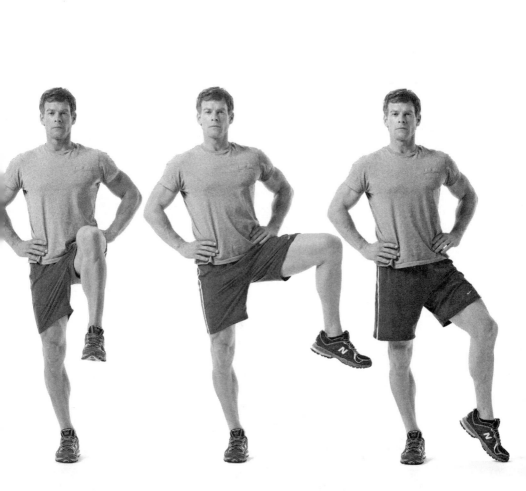

HIP CIRCLE
Stand with your feet together and your hands resting on your hips. Lift your left leg up, bending your knee to 90 degrees. Rotate the hip out to the side and back, then lower. Next raise it back to the side and rotate it forward, then lower.
➡ **Do 10 times, then repeat the move with the right leg.**

HAMSTRING STRETCH

Lie on your back on the floor. Bend your left knee to 90 degrees, keeping that foot flat on the floor. Raise your right leg as straight as you can with help from your hands clasped around your thigh.

➡ **Hold for 30 seconds, then repeat the stretch with your left leg elevated.**

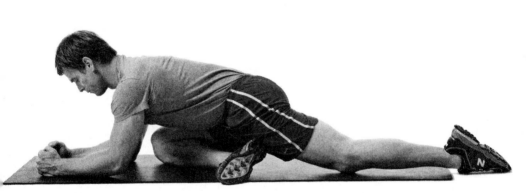

BUTT STRETCH

This move stretches the piriformis muscle found deep within the buttocks. A tight piriformis can trigger lower back pain or irritation of the nearby sciatic nerve. To do the stretch, start by getting on your hands and knees. Bring your right knee forward and move your foot across your body to the outside of your left hip. Slide the other knee back and feel the stretch in the buttocks.

➡ **Hold for 30 seconds, then repeat the stretch with the left leg.**

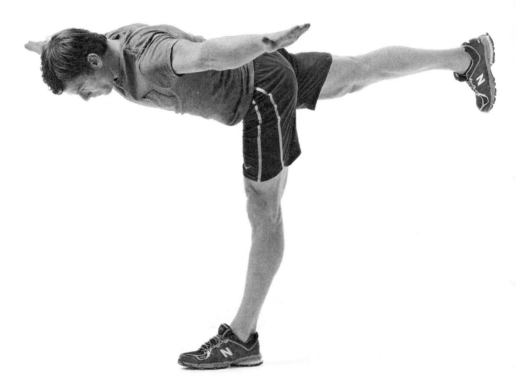

AIRPLANE

Stand with your feet together. Extend your arms out to the sides to form a T. While tightening your abdominal and lower back muscles, bend forward at the hips, simultaneously raising your right leg off the floor behind you. Try forming a straight line with your back and leg.

➡ **Hold for 10 seconds, 5 times. Then repeat this dynamic stretch with the left leg.**

BACK LUNGE AND TWIST

Start with your feet together. Step back with your right leg and bend your left knee to 90 degrees. Twist your trunk to the left, extending your arms to deepen the stretch.

➡ **Do a total of 10 repetitions, then do the back lunge with your left leg.**

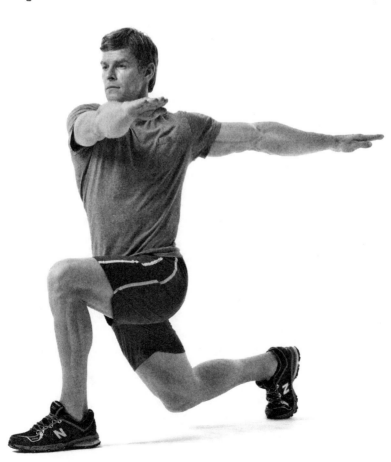

BUTTERFLY STRETCH

This stretch releases the groin muscle, inner thighs, and hip flexor. Sit on the floor, put the soles of your feet together and bend at the knees, making a diamond with your legs. Bring your heels toward your groin, lowering your knees toward the floor and slowly bring your chest toward the ground.

➡ **Hold the stretch for 15 to 30 seconds. Relax and repeat several times.**

TIP: **For a greater challenge, bring your feet closer to the glutes.**

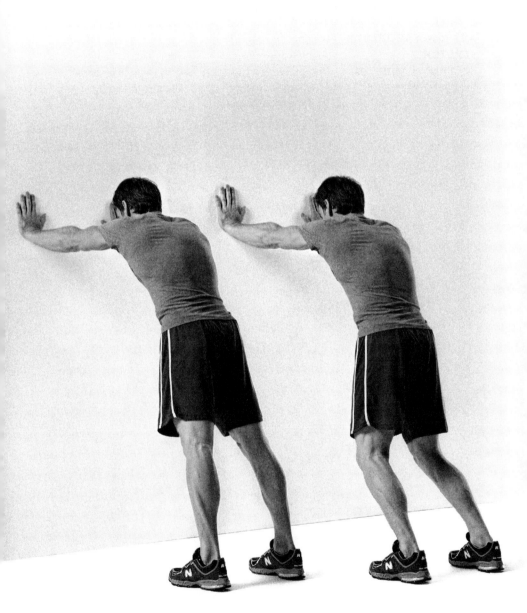

CALF STRETCH

Keeping your calves flexible will help you avoid Achilles tendonitis and calf tears. Stand about 3 feet from a wall with your feet about shoulder-width apart. Lean into the wall with your hands against it while keeping your legs straight and your heels on the floor. You'll feel the stretch in the backs of the calves.
➡ **Hold for 30 seconds, rest, and repeat, this time with your knees slightly bent.**

ANTERIOR SHOULDER STRETCH
Place your left arm across the front of your body above your chest. With the opposite hand, grasp your elbow.
Now pull your arm across your body (without twisting your torso) until you feel tension in your deltoid and chest.
➡ **Hold for 15 seconds
Perform five with each arm.**

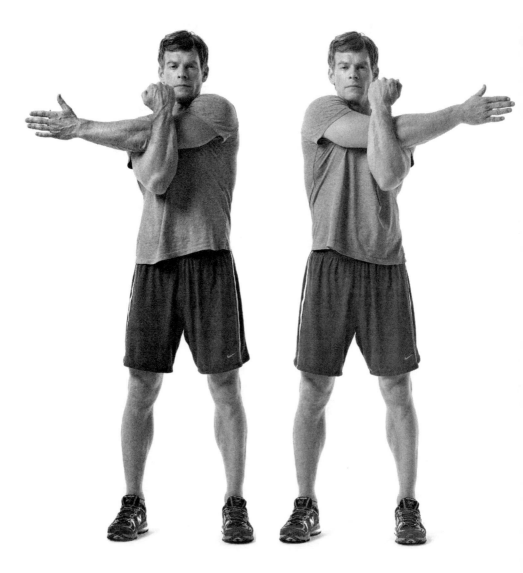

Speed Stretch
No time to stretch? Here's a total-body quickie

Sometimes your window-of-workout opportunity is tiny and you may be tempted to go headlong into your training without a warmup or stretch. Don't do it. Don't skip stretching. It's the best thing you can do to prevent injury.

Here's an option for you, a combination move called the **Forward Lunge, Elbow to Instep**. It stretches nearly every muscle in the body, says performance coach Mark Verstegen. It also creates symmetrical strength and stability, which helps boost athletic performance. But before you do this dynamic stretch, we recommend warming up your muscles a bit by walking around or running in place. Ready?

Step forward with your right leg, as if doing a traditional lunge, and place your left hand on the floor. Move your right elbow to

your right instep; hold for two seconds. Next, place your right hand on the ground next to your right instep, and rotate your left arm and chest toward the sky; hold for 2 seconds. Place your left hand on the floor, move your right

hand to the outside of your right foot, and push your hips toward the sky, pulling your right toe toward your right shin. Step forward into the next lunge with your left foot and repeat the stretch on your left side.

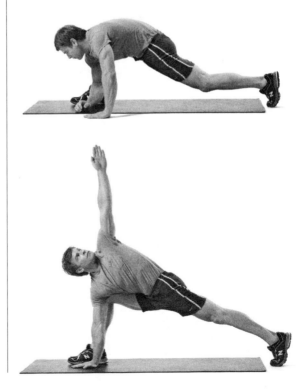

STRESS LESS, SLEEP BETTER

The Fit 40+ Body
Needs to Relax, Keep Cool, and Sleep Deeply

Tump-bump, bump-bump, bump-bump . . .
It's three in the morning, and you're lying in bed feverishly reviewing revenue projections and head counts, fighting off the premonition of someone being handed a pink slip—maybe someone from your division, maybe your supervisor, maybe you. The only thing is, once you've started, now you can't turn off the worry. Your pulse is so loud it bangs in your ears. Six hours from now the interdepartmental meeting begins, and you have no idea what to expect: promotion or reorganization? Sleep would help.

Yeah, right.

You get up and pour yourself some warm milk. You take deep relaxation breaths and count sheep backward from 100. Nothing works, and now your worries multiply, as other pressures of the fortysomething life grab your conscious mind—your humbled stock portfolio, your parents' ages, and your 16-year-old daughter's ➡

latest boyfriend who goes by a single name—Skull.

This is modern stress in all its painful glory. All those nebulous nighttime fears—the job, the retirement fund, the inmate, *er*, boyfriend—trigger the same physiological response that kept our ancient ancestors on their toes when a giant mastodon appeared in their paths. Known as the "fight or flight response," it's the same physical reaction that blasts adrenaline through your body when your neighbor's German shepherd starts nipping at your running shorts. No wonder you're still awake.

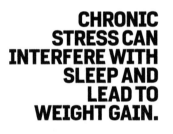

CHRONIC STRESS CAN INTERFERE WITH SLEEP AND LEAD TO WEIGHT GAIN.

The hub of all this action is a piece of your primal brain called the *amygdala*. Stemming from the Greek word for almond, this nut-shaped structure (actually it's two almond-like structures) resides on each side of your brain atop the brainstem. The amygdala is a vault for your emotional memory and central station for your body's response to fear. Emotions are hard-wired, biological functions of the nervous system that evolved to help animals survive in hostile environments, says Joseph LeDoux, PhD, a neuroscientist at New York University, pioneer of amygdala research, and author of the book,

The Emotional Brain. "The things that make rats and people afraid are very different," says LeDoux, "but the way the brain deals with danger appears to be similar."

With the speed of a tripwire, the amygdala reacts instantaneously to a perceived threat—the bark of that dog or the sound of your boss's voice. The amygdala and its neural connections at the center of the limbic brain commandeer every part of your gray matter to deal with crisis. One of those areas is the hypothalamus, which secretes corticotropin-releasing hormone (the body's emergency-response substance), which activates the sympathetic nervous system: Blood rushes to the large muscles of the limbs to prepare for flight, pupils dilate, heart rate and respiration accelerate, and digestive activity slows to send more blood to the limbs. The neurotransmitter dopamine floods the brain to rivet your attention on the source of the fear. But what does all that mean?

"For 99 percent of the beasts on this planet, stress is about three minutes of screaming terror as you sprint for your life on the savanna, after which it's either over with, or you're over with," says Robert Sapolsky, PhD, a professor of biology and neurology at the Stanford University School of Medicine and the author of *Why Zebras Don't Get Ulcers.*

We humans rarely face short-term, sharp-toothed stress. There just aren't that many opportunities to be surprised by a hungry lion in the well-groomed suburb of Maplewood. Instead, our fears take a different form—that of recurring thoughts about the future.

Obsessive worry can affect your reasoning and cognition and even paralyze your mind's critical abilities. Short-term memory, creativity, and planning functions evaporate from the obsessed, stressed human brain. With this primal-fear response turned on indefinitely, some sink into chronic anxiety, panic, or depression. According to the Public Health Service, about 50 percent of mental problems reported in the United States are anxiety disorders, and most of those are related to the brain's fear system, says LeDoux. Chronic stress can also lead to weight gain and abdominal fat [see How Stress Makes You Fat, page 154]. It can disrupt the body's metabolism, causing blood sugar to rise, triggering cells to store fat, contributing to muscle breakdown, and instigating appetite and cravings. Investigations by researchers in Italy show that stress stimulates cravings particularly for fatty and starchy foods. A similar study at Yale University found that people with higher levels of the stress hormone cortisol (more on that later) in their blood ate more food, especially sweets, than people with lower cortisol levels.

Stress's most visible side effect may be abdominal fat, but it also plays a more covert role in your health—by compromising the power of your immune system. In a study at the Ohio State University College of Medicine, researchers administered small puncture wounds to a group of dental school students at two different times: once during exams and again during a vacation period. When the scientists examined how the wounds healed, they found that all the students took three days longer, on average, to heal during the stressful exams than during the vacation break. The reason? Stress may inhibit tissue-repairing cells in our bloodstreams.

STRESS PLAYS A MORE COVERT ROLE IN YOUR HEALTH— COMPROMISING YOUR IMMUNE SYSTEM.

Think about the last time you caught a cold virus. Chances are it happened while you were under stress or simply exhausted at the time. Research from Carnegie Mellon University in Pittsburgh found that undergoing severe stress for more than a month doubled a person's risk for catching a cold. "Certain stressful life events that are chronic and enduring, such as poor marriages or unsatisfying jobs, appear to have a connection," says Sheldon Cohen, PhD, a professor of psychology at Carnegie Mellon University. "Happy, enthusiastic people are less susceptible to colds."

Stress has been linked to more serious ailments than the common cold—heart disease, high blood pressure, stroke, cancer, and sexual disorders. Up to 90 percent of all visits to doctors in the United States are for stress-related disorders, according to the American Institute of Stress.

Self-Test: How Stressed Are You?

For a quick picture of your stress profile, check your responses to the following statements and compare your score to the key below

Q. IN THE PAST MONTH, HOW OFTEN HAVE YOU...

➡ Felt you could handle your personal challenges?

___ Very often
___ Fairly often
___ Sometimes
___ Almost never
___ Never

➡ Felt that, in general, things were going your way?

___ Very often
___ Fairly often
___ Sometimes
___ Almost never
___ Never

➡ Been able to cope with all the things you had to do?

___ Very often
___ Fairly often
___ Sometimes
___ Almost never
___ Never

➡ Been able to control your irritation with situations in your life?

___ Very often
___ Fairly often
___ Sometimes
___ Almost never
___ Never

➡ Had a good night's sleep?

___ Very often
___ Fairly often
___ Sometimes
___ Almost never
___ Never

SCORING

Give yourself
0 points for each "very often,"
1 for each "fairly often,"
2 for each "sometimes,"
3 for each "almost never," and
4 for each "never."

0 TO 3 POINTS Your easygoing mentality allows you to take stress in stride.

4 TO 7 POINTS You're in control most of the time, but cracks are starting to show.

8 TO 11 POINTS Try the stress-reduction techniques starting on page 152. And work out for 30 minutes a day, 3 days a week.

12 POINTS OR MORE Your stress levels are high. Consider talking to a counselor or mental-health professional.

And as you are well aware, stress often comes between you and a good night's sleep. For that, you can thank your glucocorticoids.

Glucocorticoids are steroid hormone molecules—cortisol and adrenaline—that are secreted by your adrenal glands into your bloodstream during times of stress. They help shuttle energy into your limbs, and they enhance the connections between neurons in the brain's hippocampus. They keep you all jazzed up. During the slow-wave stages of deep, restful sleep, however, your stress response is turned off. Glucocorticoid secretion powers down deep in the night, until about an hour before you wake up, and presto, you awaken refreshed.

That's the way it's supposed to work. But when you are under stress, or sleep deprived, glucocorticoid secretion and your sympathetic nervous system become activated at the wrong times. That stress causes more glucocorticoids in your brain during sleep, which means you don't sleep as deeply and you don't get the same level of energy rejuvenation. You wake up sleep-deprived, which has the same effect as other kinds of stress—it keeps your brain full of glucocorticoids, making it hard to sleep the next night, and so on and so on.

LET'S BREAK IT DOWN: MORE STRESS = LESS QUALITY SLEEP = AN OLDER BRAIN.

Nodding off during your boss's presentation isn't the only danger here. Laboratory evidence suggests that prolonged levels of elevated glucocorticoid can cause the connections between neurons in the hippocampus to shrivel. One study measured a 14-percent smaller hippocampal volume in chronically stressed people who had elevated levels of cortisol in their bloodstreams compared to people who had normal levels of the stress hormone. The scientists at the Douglas Research Centre in Quebec also found that the stressed-out folks performed worse on memory tests than did those with normal cortisol.

Let's break it down: more stress = less quality sleep = an older brain. Time to make some changes.

De-Stress: The Road to a Good Night's Sleep

It is estimated that three out of four cases of insomnia are instigated by stress. But remember, it's not the stressors themselves, but how we handle them: One survey of stressed-out adults found that 57 percent stop exercising when they are under stress and 46 percent don't care much about what they eat. If you want to control your stress, you'll be much more successful if you fuel your body properly and exercise every day.

Exercise builds confidence and a feeling of self-mastery that's a powerful coping mechanism. Kicking a friend's butt in a tennis match gives you a sense of accomplishment. So does biking 20 miles. And it's nearly impossible to dwell on your worries when you are doing the American crawl in a swimming pool. You'll be too busy trying to breathe! Exercising is a terrific distraction to shift your focus away from negative thoughts.

One study at the University of Texas Southwestern Medical Center showed that regular aerobic exercise was as effective as antidepressant medication at treating mild clinical depression. Exercise pumps up the mood-regulating neurotransmitter serotonin as well as the feel-good chemicals norepinephrine, dopamine, and endorphins. Exercise also triggers cells to release peptides that increase body temperature. "Working out has a calming effect similar to that of spending time in a sauna or a hot shower, and all three can help relieve anxiety and depression," says Larry Leith, PhD, author of *Exercising Your Way to Better Mental Health*. And exercise strengthens your heart, which protects it from the dangers of stress.

A body that's fit and well-fueled is more resistant to mental stress and better prepared to deal with the pressures of modern life and approach them with a healthy perspective. For the past two decades, Robert Maurer, PhD, a clinical psychologist at UCLA's School of Medicine, has treated hundreds of people suffering from anxiety by teaching them to call stress what it really is: fear.

"There are only two basic fears," says Maurer. "One is that you're not worthwhile or good enough to get the job or whatever; and the other is that you're going to lose control, such as in health or financial concerns."

In order to escape the symptoms of fear, he says, you must admit to being scared and recognize fear as the body's way of preparing itself for action. Most of us think of anxiety and fear

How Stress Makes You Fat

The mechanism that turns your fears into flab

1

STRESSOR

Divorce lawyer, overbearing boss, you name it.

➡ **HYPOTHALAMUS** responds by secreting corticotropin-releasing hormone (CRH), which travels through the capillaries to the pituitary gland.

➡ **PITUITARY GLAND** releases adrenocortico-trophic hormone (ACTH).

➡ **ADRENAL GLANDS** flood the bloodstream with two stress hormones, epinephrine (adrenaline) and cortisol.

2

ADRENALINE

Switches on the body's primordial fight-or-flight response:

➡ **HEART RATE AND PULSE** quicken to send extra blood to the muscles.

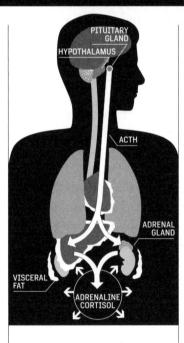

➡ **BRONCHIAL TUBES** dilate to accept extra oxygen to feed the brain and keep us alert.

➡ **BLOOD VESSELS** constrict to stem bleeding in case of an injury.

3

CORTISOL (YOUR FRIEND)

Cortisol and adrenaline release fat and sugar (glucose) into the bloodstream for use as energy to deal with the stressor in an emergency. That works perfectly during short-term stress, such as when you need to fend off the dog chasing your bike.

4

CORTISOL (YOUR ENEMY)

Cortisol can also signal your cells to store fat. This occurs when cortisol levels remain high due to long-term mental stressors. Chronically elevated cortisol disrupts the body's metabolic control systems: Muscle breaks down, blood sugar rises, appetite increases, and you get fat! What's worse, the fat tends to accumulate in the abdominal region and on the artery walls.

as something negative to avoid. But it's not a sign of weakness, says Maurer; it's a call for courage and fuel for positive change. The symptoms of fear—insomnia, stomach distress, rapid heart rate, sweating—are normal, healthy signals. When you feel them, identify your fear, and then find people who can help you deal with it. "Our culture values independence, but what your body really craves is to draw strength from others," says Maurer.

Here are some other ways to walk the fine line between healthy challenge and destructive anxiety.

+ **Create a three-legged life.** Add balance to your life—your home, your work, yourself—to create a buffer against stress. "If one goes down, you have others to hold you up," says Mounir Soliman, MD, director of the Center for Wellness & Personal Growth at the University of California, San Diego. When top executives are asked to put a percentage value on three key areas of their lives, a typical response is 40 percent work, 30 percent parenting, and 30 percent community and friends, says Soliman. "They strongly believe they are spending that much time on those values, but when you really analyze it, they may spend 70 percent of their time focused on work. That's where you find unhealthy imbalance."

+ **Plan more efficiently.** "Planning is the most important thing [you] can do to avoid stress," says psychologist Michael Kahn, PhD, who has interviewed more than 100 executives about how they handle stress. "Make a habit of reflective engagement: Check in with yourself once a day or once a week to plan ahead." he says. Sunday night is a good time to take half an hour and plan out the first few days of the week. Or do it in the morning before you open your e-mail or become bombarded by interruptions.

"I learned in the Navy that if you make a list of all the things that need to be done, you get them out of your head and you don't have to think about them," says one of Kahn's clients. "When I have too much on the plate, the only way I can gain a sense of control is to put them in a sequence of priority, the old A-B-C theory. You know, the As need to be done. The Bs ought to be done. The Cs can wait."

+ **Learn how to say no.** Someone who has too much on his plate needs to be able to say no to more without regret. That's where good planning can help. Schedule regular appointments into your week—like a Wednesday tennis lesson—so that you are not always reacting to others' needs. And learn to delegate. A good manager will always look to relinquish tasks that others can do, so that he can focus on things only he can do. People who are perpetually stressed at work are often perfectionists, who feel that no one can do the job as well as they can, so they try to do everything and end up undermining their performance.

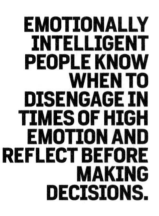

EMOTIONALLY INTELLIGENT PEOPLE KNOW WHEN TO DISENGAGE IN TIMES OF HIGH EMOTION AND REFLECT BEFORE MAKING DECISIONS.

+ **Call a time-out.** You expend a lot of emotional energy in a reactive mode. When you feel a tide of anger or frustration rising in you, call a time-out and leave the room to regain your composure. Just as a basketball coach will call a time-out to slow down the pace of the game and regroup when the other team is on a run, emotionally intelligent people know when to disengage in times of high emotion, reflect on their core values, and recharge before making decisions.

+ **Pick off the low-hanging fruit.** Being faced with a seemingly impossible challenge can easily lead to procrastination. When you feel it happening to you, immediately pinpoint at least one piece of the problem that you can control, and attack it. When you shift into "take-charge" mode, you meet a challenge from a position of strength rather than feeling at its mercy. Often, that'll be enough to buck up your confidence and set you on a path of action.

+ **Turn trouble into transformation.** In 1929, some men were so consumed with their financial problems that they jumped out of buildings. "Yet there were people who walked away from the terror of the Holocaust, chose to move ahead without a penny, and succeeded," says Mel Schwartz, a Westport, Connecticut-based psychotherapist. "A crisis is an opportunity to escape programmed living and transform yourself. The more creative and participatory you feel when forced outside of your comfort zone, the more balanced and happy you will ultimately be."

+ **Focus on somebody besides numero uno.** Our preoccupation with comparing ourselves to our friends and rivals can easily get us into mental health trouble. "People who have a problem with anxiety often get lost in measuring and judging themselves," says Schwartz. "It's a very Newtonian worldview. We measure to create order in our lives and in doing so we lose our humanity and our connection to one another. The critical voice is enslaving."

Try focusing on others. Showing respect and appreciation for others has an amazing ability to diffuse obsessive behavior and anxiety caused by preoccupation with the self. Volunteer at a soup kitchen. Teach illiterate folks how to read. Mentor a teenager at your place of worship or at the local high school. Helping others will give you a sense of self-respect, and engaging with others will break the isolation that magnifies your worries. Plus, helping others offers another worthwhile benefit: It may help you to live longer. Studies show that people who volunteer their time at least once a week regularly outlive those who don't do volunteer work.

+ **Stomp on the ANTs.** To escape the grip of self-doubt you have to recognize the ANTs—Automatic Negative Thoughts. ANTs give you a constant glass-half-empty view of your life situation. When you are always choosing the doomsday scenario, you need to check yourself. "Simply identifying negativity as ANTs can help you gain control over them," says psychologist and leadership expert Mario Alonso, PhD. Use humor to take your fears to the extreme by asking yourself, "Am I really going to end up dumpster diving for my dinner?" Also, disassociate yourself from negative thoughts by learning to observe them but not react.

+ **Stop trying to multitask.** You respond to e-mail while talking to someone on the phone. You try to read the paper while watching TV and playing with your kids. You attempt to juggle three different projects at once and promise to get three tasks done by the end of the day when, realistically, there's time to accomplish just one. With more and more pressure to produce, you try to squeeze more out of the little time you have. Yet while multitasking may seem more efficient on the surface, study after study shows that you don't gain anything but more stress by trying to do two or three tasks at once.

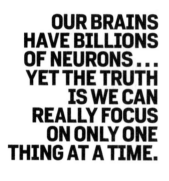

OUR BRAINS HAVE BILLIONS OF NEURONS... YET THE TRUTH IS WE CAN REALLY FOCUS ON ONLY ONE THING AT A TIME.

"Our brains have billions of neurons, each making thousands of connections, and yet the truth is we can really focus on only one thing at a time," says Rene Marois, PhD, a neuroscientist and associate professor of psychology at Vanderbilt University, who has studied the brains of people trying to do two tasks at once. The brain scans reveal an actual neural bottleneck in our frontal lobes, where executive functions such as decision-making and memory occur. Try to accomplish two things at once, and you invariably slow down or mess up. This is why someone on the other end of the phone can always tell from your distracted tone of voice that you're checking e-mail.

A study in the *Journal of Experimental Psychology* measured the speed with which subjects switched between two different tasks, one solving math problems and another classifying geometric objects, in four experiments of varying degrees of complexity. The measurements for all the experiments showed that participants lost time when they had to switch from one task to another rather than complete one task before moving on to the next. In addition, the subjects took significantly longer to switch when either the tasks became much more difficult or they switched between very different types of tasks. That's why it's so difficult to get back to writing a detailed report when someone pops into your office to chat.

Dave Crenshaw, author of the book *The Myth of Multitasking*, says a person can do two things at once effectively as long as long as the tasks don't require much attention. "Background tasking, doing something mindless and mundane like watching TV while running on a treadmill, is actually pretty efficient," he says. But multitasking, or *switchtasking* as he prefers to call it, never is. By toggling back and forth between tasks, people lose time; it's far less productive, he says. Try this adaptation of an exercise Crenshaw uses in talks to make his point. Time yourself while writing the sentence "This is taking much too long." Each time you write one of the letters in each word, write a number, starting with 1, below it. So, you'll write T, then 1 below it; H, then 2 below it; and so on. Your paper will look like this:

```
T  H  I  S  I  S  T  A  K  I  N  G  M  U  C  H  T  O  O  L  O  N  G
1  2  3  4  5  6  7  8  9  10 11 12 13 14 15 16 17 18 19 20 21 22 23
```

Now time yourself while writing the sentence straight through and then numbers 1 through 23 consecutively, without switching between the two tasks. You'll find you do the second exercise much quicker. That's because your brain slows down when switching between tasks but uses the power of momentum to zip through each single task. "When you switchtask on a computer, you simply lose efficiency," says Crenshaw. Switchtask on your wife, husband, or boss, and you'll exponentially add to your stress level. "It can be very hurtful to the relationship," he says. "Be present, listen carefully, and make sure everything has been taken care of before moving on."

+ **Beware of e-mail addiction.** As much as modern technology may streamline life, it also adds to your stress, as anyone knows who has spent an hour on the phone with tech support for help with setting up their wireless network. But you need to be able to check your e-mail outside on the deck! How many times a day do you check it on your computer or BlackBerry? Often

Chill Drill
Try this stress management ritual

1

Recognize your mind–body signals of distress— muscle tensions, rapid pulse, sweaty palms, and obsessive worry.

2

Disengage with a walk or this mind-centering breathing exercise: Breathe deeply through your nose so that your belly rises before your chest does and exhale through your mouth.

3

Identify the source of the stress—a project, a deadline, a personal interaction.

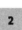 **4**

Generate a realistic solution that you can implement

immediately. For example, you might recognize that "I am trying to do 2 days worth of tasks in 4 hours!" The solution might be to decide to postpone doing one item on your list and save it for another time.

what keeps you checking in is the fear that you'll miss something important from a colleague or supervisor. Tom Stafford, PhD, a cognitive neuroscientist at the University of Sheffield in Britain, believes that e-mail addiction is classic psychological behaviorism. You may recall from Psych 101 that the best way to reinforce a behavior is to reward it—not always, but occasionally, at random times. So, if you want your golden retriever to bring you your slippers, you give him a treat when he does it right. Not every time; you want to keep him guessing. The same thing works with us and e-mail. We'll check it 20 times a day because every so often we'll get good news or receive positive reinforcement. We e-mail addicts are just a bunch of dogs salivating for Liv-A Snaps!

+ **Heal yourself with acupressure.** Next time you're feeling tense, give yourself a hand. Acupressure is a quick tension releaser, according to researchers at Hong Kong Polytechnic University who found it can reduce stress by up to 39 percent. For fast relief, massage the fleshy part between the thumb and index finger for 20 to 30 seconds. This is a universal pressure point for easing upper-body tension, according to the American Physical Therapy Association. Simply stretching in your office can trigger feelings of calm, as well. A study in the *American Journal of Industrial Medicine* found that office workers who took a 15-minute stretch break felt calmer and more productive afterward. Try these desk stretches when you feel the grip of stress in your neck and back.

➡ **THORACIC FLEX.** With hands behind your head, bend your upper body over your chair's back as far as possible. Draw your shoulder blades together, and hold for 2 seconds. Release, and repeat 8 times.

➡ **HIP-FLEXORS STRETCH.** Place a foot on a stable chair or step and lean forward while extending your arms overhead. Gently arch your back while moving your arms (keep 'em straight) back slightly. Hold for 2 seconds. Release, and repeat 8 times. (For more terrific stress-busting at-work stretches, see Chapter 5.)

+ **Respect the power of your imagination.** When people worry, they tend to build a story in their minds to perpetuate their fears. That's where self-awareness can help. If you recognize yourself doing it, you can hit the brakes.

+ **Respect the unexpected.** Kahn says that efficient executives tend to be very sensitive to the feeling of becoming overwhelmed; when they recognize it happening, they take action. "'I'm in this job 24/7,' one company president told me," says Kahn. 'If I don't handle stress well, I'm not going to perform well or last very long.'"

Learn to Sleep Like a Baby in Your 40s

Every couple who shares a bed knows there are differences between women and men when it comes to sleep patterns. Men generally develop sleep problems in their 30s and 40s, usually in reaction to situations out of their control. Women, on the other hand, can have difficulty sleeping during the pre- and postmenopausal periods due to changes in hormones. Pregnancy wreaks havoc on sleep patterns, especially during the last few weeks. Postpartum, some women may struggle with falling to sleep for days, even weeks, and it may have nothing to do with the blood-curdling screams emanating from the little angel in the nursery.

Insomnia can be triggered by dozens of mental, physical, and environmental causes. We've already made our point about fear as the key instigator of sleepless nights, worry, tension, anxiety, and depression. Other common instigators are pain; illness; snoring and sleep apnea; indigestion; stimulants like caffeine and chocolate; and foods like cookies, candy, and cakes that can cause blood-sugar spikes. Alcohol, which is a depressant, can have a stimulating effect that keeps you up, and it certainly is known to disrupt deep restful sleep even without the bed spins. Even doing something as good for you as exercising can make it difficult to fall asleep, if you do it late enough, by stimulating your adrenal levels and energizing your muscles.

So, if you aren't sure why you're not getting a good night of restful sleep, you'll probably have to do a little detective work to identify your sleep gremlins. What is very clear is that sleep is immensely important to good health. Sleep shuts down your body so it can repair and rebuild. During sleep, your body releases its greatest concentration of growth hormone—the substance that helps strengthen damaged tissue. Sleep also provides an opportunity to heal your mind by allowing your brain to relax. Skimping on sleep can lead to nodding off behind the wheel on your morning commute. It can dim your brainpower and affect your career if not addressed.

Studies have also shown a close connection between disrupted sleep and a compromised immune system. When do you typically catch the common cold? When you're stressed and sleep-deprived. What's the best remedy for the common cold besides grandma's chicken soup? It's sleep.

Sleeplessness can also cause you to put on belly fat and elevate your risk for heart attack and diabetes. Indeed, clinical research shows that blood pressure and heart rate increase when people are denied shut-eye. "Some research has suggested that sleep restriction over many years may affect metabolism, increasing the risk of obesity and type 2 diabetes," says Siobhan Banks, PhD, an assistant professor of psychiatry at the University of Pennsylvania. In fact, a 2007 Canadian study found that people who sleep only 5 to 6 hours a night increase their likelihood of being overweight by 69 percent, compared with those who habitually sleep 7 to 8 hours.

A study at the University of Chicago suggests why: It found a correlation between sleep and two hunger hormones—ghrelin, which triggers you to eat, and leptin, which tells you you're full. The researchers limited 12 young men to 4 hours sleep on two consecutive nights, then measured their hunger hormones afterward. The eating accelerator ghrelin was up 28 percent, while the I've-had-enough hormone leptin was down 18 percent. Another study at Baruch College in New York City found that daytime drowsiness triggers cravings for unhealthy foods.

It doesn't take much to dip into a sleep deficit. Sleep doctors say that missing just 1 hour of sleep on 7 consecutive nights has the same physiological effect as staying awake for 24 hours straight. The optimum number of hours of sleep for good health is 8, according to the National Sleep Foundation, yet Americans are sleeping on average only about 6.9 hours. More than 18 million Americans suffer from one or more of the 70 different types of chronic sleep disorders, says the National Commission on Sleep Disorders Research. The long nights of cramming for exams may be long gone, but sleepless nights can increase as you get older. During your 30s and 40s, you may get as much as 82 percent less deep, "slow-wave" sleep than you did in your teens and 20s. Slow-wave sleep is the important regenerative sleep your body needs to rebuild itself.

Take the quiz on page 170 to determine if you can count yourself among the walking dead-tired. If you are, try some of the techniques, in this chapter, to pinpoint your sleep-

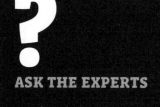

ASK THE EXPERTS

Q. What do you do to relieve stress?
I listen to chill-out music. I like the Buddha Bar CDs
and the Chillout Lounge channel on 1Club.FM, a free
Internet radio station.

— P. MURALI DORAISWAMY, MD,
chief of the biological psychiatry division at Duke University

disturbing triggers and prepare yourself for a better night's rest.
The good news is that 8 hours of good quality sleep are all you
need to usher you back into the world of wakefulness, as if you
have been sleeping like a baby all week.

When you sleep better, you'll feel better. Understanding just
how sleep happens and why it's so important may help you to
get better sleep or at least convince you to DVR *Late Night with
David Letterman* instead of staying up.

The Stages of Sleep

As you go through your busy day, a chemical messenger called
adenosine builds up in your body. This neurotransmitter is
created as your body burns through glucose to energize your
actions. The more adenosine builds up in your brain, the sleep-
ier you will feel. This is one reason people who exercise sleep
better. They burn more glucose and therefore store up more
adenosine. At the same time this stuff is making your brain
fuzzy, another brain chemical, melatonin, is being secreted. Its
release is cued by your internal circadian clock, which is sensitive to light and time of day. As the evening wanes and darkness
falls, more melatonin floods your brain to power you down and
make you yawn. When you fall asleep, you alternate between
deep restorative sleep and more alert stages and dream sleep.
Your unconscious journey through the night is made up of

stages, reflecting the pattern of electrical waves in the sleeping mind. There are two basic states of the sleep cycle: rapid eye movement (REM) and non-rapid eye-movement (NREM) sleep, the latter consisting of stages 1 through 4. During an average night, you typically experience four or five complete cycles.

Stage 1 is very brief, lasting just 5 or 10 minutes. In this stage, your eyes move slowly under your eyelids, your body starts to slow down, but you are just drowsy.

In stage 2, light sleep, your eyes stop moving, your heart rate slows, and your body temperature decreases. But if your toddler cries out for a glass of water or your dog barks at a prowler, you'll still spring out of bed easily to deal with the crisis.

Next comes the deep sleep of stages 3 and 4 when it's very difficult to rouse you from slumber. This is when your brain gets its rest. In stage 4 your body secretes growth hormone to repair and restore your muscles. It is also thought to be the time that immune functions increase.

About an hour and a half into the sleep cycle, you drift into REM sleep. Breathing speeds up, heart rate increases, and blood pressure rises. This is when guys get erections and women experience their equivalent clitoral enlargement, and your brain is writing bizzare screenplays involving long-ago lovers, hula hoops, and fox terriers that play the ukulele. Dream sleep is essential to our brains for processing memories, emotions, and stress. Researchers believe dreaming allows crucial learning and skill building.

The experts say that hitting a snooze alarm over and over to wake up is not the best way to feel rested. "The restorative value of rest is diminished, especially when the increments are short," said psychologist Edward Stepanski, PhD, who has studied sleep fragmentation at the Rush University Medical Center in Chicago. This on-and-off-again effect of dozing and waking causes shifts in the brain-wave patterns. Sleep-deprived snooze-button addicts are likely to shorten their quota of REM sleep, impairing their mental functioning during the day.

Certain therapies, like cognitive behavioral therapy, teach people how to recognize and change patterns of thought and behavior to solve their problems. Recently this type of therapy has been shown to be very effective in getting people to fall asleep and conquer insomnia.

How to Get Optimum, Restful Sleep

+ **Deal with your stress.** If stress is keeping you up at night, working with a therapist to get to the root of your anxiety is a good bet. According to a study published in the *Archives of Internal Medicine,* cognitive behavior therapy is more effective and lasts longer than the widely used sleeping pill, Ambien, in reducing insomnia. In the study, 63 people with insomnia were given Ambien, cognitive behavior therapy, both, or a placebo. The patients in the therapy group were given daily exercises to recognize, challenge, and change stress-inducing thoughts; and were taught to get out of bed and read if, after 20 minutes of trying, they were having trouble falling asleep. After 3 weeks, 44 percent of the patients receiving the cognitive therapy and those receiving the combination therapy and pills fell asleep faster, compared to 29 percent of the patients taking only the sleeping pills. Two weeks after the treatment was completed, all the patients in the therapy group were able to fall asleep in half the time it took them before beginning the study. Only 17 percent of the patients taking sleeping pills fell asleep in half the time. For an immediate remedy for your overactive mind, get up and walk to another part of the house. (Keep the lights off to avoid triggering your brain to wake up.) Often your anxious thoughts will stop, and you can return to your room to go to sleep. This strategy, called stimulus control, also prevents you from associating your bed with anxiety.

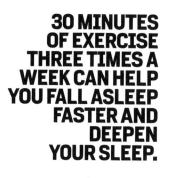

30 MINUTES OF EXERCISE THREE TIMES A WEEK CAN HELP YOU FALL ASLEEP FASTER AND DEEPEN YOUR SLEEP.

+ **Break a sweat.** The National Sleep Foundation reports that 30 minutes of exercise, three or more times a week, can help you fall asleep faster and deepen your sleep. *When* you exercise can have an impact, too. University of Arizona researchers say that working out late in the afternoon is best because the natural dip in body temperature 5 to 6 hours after you exercise may make you drowsy before bedtime. Whatever time you choose to work out, be wary of exercising too close to bedtime, which can actually make it harder to fall asleep.

+ **Bore your brain.** If you have racing thoughts, sometimes jotting what's on your mind onto a piece of paper will help you get it out of your head, especially if it's something important that you don't want to forget. More likely, however, runaway worries are keeping you from falling asleep. Here are three tricks to try.

➡ **WRITE NEGATIVES.** If you are catastrophizing, that is, worrying about things that may happen, write down the worst-case scenario. That may help you to realize that you are worrying about "what ifs" that may never even happen, and that even if they do happen, it won't be the end of the world. Often, that's enough to break the cycle of worry.

➡ **READ A BOOK.** The old-school insomniac's cure really works. The repetition of reading lines in a book tires the eyes and helps your brain relax, says Alex Chediak, MD, medical director of the Miami Sleep Disorders Center.

➡ **CHALLENGE YOURSELF.** Equally effective ways to bore your brain into slumber: crossword puzzles and counting backward by threes. Counting forces you to concentrate on something other than your racing thoughts. "It's hard and so boring, you'll fall right asleep," says sleep specialist Michael Breus, PhD, author of *Good Night.*

+ **Hit the sack on a regular schedule.** Many sleep experts say one of the best things you can do to improve your sleep is to maintain a regular sleep-and-wakeup schedule, and that goes for weekends as well. If you regularly go to bed around 10:30 but stay up until 11:30 on weekends, try to get up at the same time you do on the weekdays. If you sleep in an extra hour, your circadian rhythms

will be an hour behind. And be wary of naps. Keep them short—
10 to 20 minutes—and never nap in the evening. Sara Mednick,
PhD, author of *Take a Nap! Change Your Life*, recommends at
least a 3-hour buffer between your nap and your regular bedtime.
Anything closer may make it more difficult to get to sleep.

+ **Watch out for hidden caffeine.** You don't have to drink
an espresso to get a jolt of caffeine. It's in colas, tea, chocolate,
energy drinks, even protein bars. Caffeine activates stress hormones, boosts alertness, revs up heart rate and blood pressure—
the perfect storm for insomnia. Some people become more
sensitive to caffeine in their 40s. Their bodies may need more
time to break it down. And, for women, estrogen may delay
caffeine metabolism even more. During ovulation and menstrua-
tion, women take about 25 percent longer to metabolize caffeine.
To be safe, avoid caffeinated beverages and foods after 1 PM.

+ **Eat early; keep it light.** A slice of pepperoni pizza or Buffalo
wings wouldn't be wise choices before bedtime. Heavy, fatty,
spicy foods will keep you up if you eat them within 3 hours of
trying to snooze. If you're hungry, eat complex carbohydrates
like a little oatmeal or whole-grain pasta. They stimulate the
release of calming serotonin. Warm milk works, too. If you
want to stay away from carbs, try a high-protein bedtime snack
such as a small serving of cheese or milk or a hard-boiled egg.
Protein actually produces greater satiety than carbohydrates
and fat.

+ **Turn the lights down.** If you work in an office with fluorescent
lights, you might try turning them off and using desk lamps
instead. Fluorescent light may interfere with quality sleep even
if you're exposed to it hours before you go to sleep. In a Swiss
study, eight men sat under a blue light (similar to fluorescent
light) for 2 hours, stopping roughly 1 hour and 45 minutes
before bed. A sleep analysis showed that these men logged half
as much REM sleep as a group not exposed to blue light. "Blue
light suppresses melatonin, the hormone responsible for regulat-

ing sleep," says James Maas, PhD, a sleep expert at Cornell University. Artificial light from computer and television screens can also be interpreted by your brain as daylight, which prevents release of this sleep-inducing chemical. For the same reason, keep your cell phone and Blackberry out of your bedroom, and turn your alarm clock away from you. Even the "blue light" from digital displays can signal your brain to wake up.

+ **Trade rubdowns with a partner.** A study in the journal *Psychosomatic Medicine* confirms what you already know from experience: Getting a back massage lowers stress, releases tension, and can help ease you into sleep mode. In the study, women who got a 30-minute massage from their husbands three times a week for a month had nearly twice the levels of the hormone oxytocin as women who didn't benefit from a rubdown. The researchers also measured an 8 percent decrease in levels of the hormone alpha-amylase, a signal of stress. Affectionate touch boosts mood and eases stress, says study author Julianne Holt-Lunstad, PhD. Sex works, too. And if one thing leads to another, post-intercourse, the body releases oxytocin, which is a nearly fail-proof sleep inducer.

+ **Sniff this herb.** In a study, 31 men and women sniffed essential oil of lavender one night and distilled water the next night just before their bedtime. Then the researchers monitored their sleep cycles with brain scans. The scans showed increased slow-wave sleep during the nights when the subjects sniffed the herb. Slow-wave sleep is the restorative sleep when heart rate slows and muscles relax. Indeed, the subjects slept more soundly and awoke feeling more energetic on the nights when they slept to the scent of lavender versus no scent at all. You can buy pure lavender essential oil at health food stores. Put a few drops on a piece of tissue and tuck it under your pillow, or use an aromatherapy diffuser.

+ **Give your legs a rest.** Restless leg syndrome (RLS) is a neurological disorder whose sensations are described by sufferers as

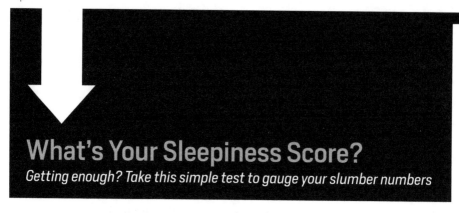

What's Your Sleepiness Score?

Getting enough? Take this simple test to gauge your slumber numbers

HOW LIKELY ARE YOU TO DOZE OFF OR FALL ASLEEP IN THE FOLLOWING SITUATIONS?

0 = no chance of dozing **1** = slight chance of dozing **2** = good chance of dozing **3** = zzzzzzzzz

_____ **Hearing a sermon at church**

_____ **Riding in a car for an hour listening to NPR**

_____ **Watching a baseball game**

_____ **Sitting and talking to your spouse**

_____ **Sitting and reading**

SCORECARD

1—6 Congrats. You're getting enough sleep or drinking a lot of coffee.

7—8 Average. You probably need to get to bed earlier.

9 AND UP Wake up and seek the counsel of a sleep specialist.

* ADAPTED FROM THE EPWORTH SLEEPINESS SCALE

ants crawling inside the legs. It's characterized by an uncontrollable urge to kick and move the legs when lying down at rest, and it is severely disruptive to sleep, causing exhaustion and daytime fatigue. Studies show that eliminating caffeine, alcohol, and tobacco may reduce symptoms. Some people find that maintaining a regular sleep schedule and moderate exercise program will help them sleep better. Taking a hot bath or massaging the lower extremities may also help soothe the savage muscle fiber. If your bed partner isn't a beefy-armed masseuse, take matters into your own hands. Pummel your quads, glutes, and calves on a foam roller or with the Stick, a self-massage warmup tool. While there is no cure for RLS, some sufferers find relief through prescription medications like levodopa and carbidopa used for treating Parkinson's disease. For more suggestions and support, visit the RLS Foundation at www.RLS.org.

+ **Be cool.** The National Sleep Foundation recommends keeping your room between 54° and 75°F. A cool, not cold, room makes it easier for your core temperature to drop, which is necessary for you to fall asleep. But you might want to wear socks to bed. That may seem counterproductive, however Swiss researchers found that cold feet and hands make your blood vessels constrict, which in turn cause you to retain heat and have trouble falling asleep. Warm feet and hands cause blood vessels to dilate, allowing heat to escape the body and your core temperature to drop, initiating sleep.

+ **Try a lullaby.** Researchers at Case Western Reserve University found that people who listen to music in the 60-to-80 beats-per-minute range (a close match to your resting heartbeat) before bedtime report more satisfying sleep. Create a play list that sets the perfect tempo, or make it easier on yourself: Order a two-CD classical or jazz set from www.bedtimebeats.com for $19.

+ **Upgrade your bed.** Take a cue from the best hotels. Chains such as Four Seasons, Westin, and W know that guests who sleep well tend to be repeat customers, so they have been working with mattress manufacturers to create the most comfortable sleep surface possible. Made to the exact specifications of each hotel, the beds feature more coils and cushioning than even high-end store models. And they are for sale. The best of the bunch are Westin's Heavenly Bed, Sheraton's Sweet Sleeper and Four Points Four Comfort Bed, and the Four Seasons signature mattress. If you've been sleeping on the same mattress for 8 years or more, it's probably time for a replacement. But you can also wrest a better night's sleep out of your old mattress simply by upgrading your sheets, blankets, and pillows.

→ SHEETS. Choose natural fibers, such as cotton, and avoid synthetics, which are less absorbent and comfy. As you shop, you'll come across the term "thread count." It reflects the number of threads woven into 1 square inch of material. The higher the thread count, the softer the sheet. But you can't get more than 500 threads into a square inch, so don't be fooled by marketing promises of 800- and 1000-thread count sheets.

➡ **BLANKETS.** One way to get an infant to sleep soundly is to swaddle him with tight blankets, which gives the secure sensation of still being in utero. "Using a comforter can give you that feeling again," says Gerard Lombardo, MD, director of the Sleep Disorders Center at New York Methodist Hospital. A good choice: Isotonic's Indulgence down-alternative comforter ($180, www.bedbathandbeyond.com). It's filled with hypoallergenic synthetic-down fibers that will keep you warm without baking you the way goose down can. Too warm for Miami? Try Wamsutta's Egyptian cotton weave blanket ($70, visit www.springs.com to find a retailer); the weave allows cool air to circulate through. If you're too warm, you won't sleep.

➡ **PILLOWS.** The most common mistake is using too many pillows or choosing one that's too big. You want a pillow that will keep your neck aligned with your spine, not bent so your chin is on your chest. "The more neutral your neck's position, the wider the nerve passageways running through it will open," says Mark McLaughlin, MD, a spinal surgeon at the University Medical Center at Princeton. That'll reduce the chance of neck pain and deliver more restful sleep. Try a memory foam pillow, which molds to your head and neck, keeping everything lined up as if you were standing straight. Two good ones are Select Comfort's Memory Foam Classic Pillow with GridZone technology ($90, www.selectcomfort. com) and the ClassicPillow by Tempur-Pedic ($100, www. tempurpedic.com).

+ **Watch for snore signals.** Chronic loud snoring of the Three Stooges variety could be the canary in the coal mine signaling sleep apnea, a common sleep disorder that, if left untreated, could be life threatening. *Apnea* is a Greek word meaning "without breath," and that's exactly what happens during sleep apnea—you literally stop breathing, sometimes hundreds of times during the night and often for a minute or longer. If you feel exhausted even after getting 8 hours of

Q. Do I benefit from the extra few minutes of sleep I get by hitting "snooze"?

Only if it gives you a chance to finish up a cool dream. It's unlikely that the extra 10 to 15 minutes will make a dent in your nightly sleep deficit. The desire to hit "snooze" comes from the instant reaction that drives you to shut off whatever blaring monstrosity just invaded your deep, peaceful sleep. May we suggest a more genteel alternative? Rather than scare you out of bed, a Zen alarm clock ($120, www.now-zen.com) uses a gradual series of chimes to rouse you, leaving you less groggy.

— **GERARD T. LOMBARDO, MD,** *director of the Sleep Disorders Center at New York Methodist Hospital*

sleep, ask your bed partner to observe you while you're sleeping to see if your breathing stops. Spouses who have observed their husbands or wives suffer through sleep apnea say it's pretty freaky waiting to see if he or she will start breathing again. Tough to get to sleep after that, but it's the best way to determine if there's a problem that needs the attention of a sleep doctor. If you're ambitious, or have an evil streak, you can videotape your snoring bedmate to show the doctor or play at family reunions.

Obstructive sleep apnea is usually caused by the movement of soft tissue in the rear of the throat—in effect, it collapses during sleep. It's usually worse if you have a wide, fatty neck—more tissue to constrict your airway. What happens during sleep is your muscles go into full relax mode, and the soft throat tissue flops down over your airway.

In central sleep apnea, the airway is not obstructed, but the brain fails to signal the muscles to breathe. Mixed apnea is a

The Downsides to Staying Up Late

DVR your late-night favorites. Regularly getting less than 7 or 8 hours of sleep takes its toll on your health. Here's how lack of sleep affects your body and mind

IT MAKES YOU BITCHY AND BUMMED OUT.
Sleep and mood are regulated by the same brain chemicals. So when you don't get a good night's rest, your mood takes a nosedive. The long-term risk is clinical depression, but probably only in people who are susceptible to the illness.

IT WEAKENS YOUR FLU FIGHTERS.
Here's proof: In one study, men given a flu shot after getting insufficient sleep had just half the disease-fighting antibodies 10 days after the vaccination when compared with a similar group of well-rested men who got the shots. Researchers say the first group of men failed to mount the normal immune response due to

combination of the two. Regardless of the type you have, the result is the same: Your brain needs to arouse you in order for you to resume breathing, which disrupts your slumber, causing poor-quality, fragmented sleep. Sleep apnea affects 12 million Americans, mostly overweight men over age 40, but it can occur in anyone. Losing weight can sometimes remedy the problem, because there is clearly a link between sleep apnea and weight gain. A new study from the University of Arizona College of Medicine found that people with sleep apnea tend to binge eat. Lose weight, eat less, sleep better. A more immediate fix for obstructive sleep apnea is sleeping on your side. Rolling onto your right or left can cause the throat-covering tissue to fall to the side, clearing the obstruction, says Edward Grandi, executive director of

their sleep deprivation. Other research found that people who got shoddy sleep for 10 days had elevated levels of C-reactive protein (CRP), an inflammation marker that has been linked to some autoimmune diseases and, of course, heart disease.

IT CRANKS YOUR CRAVINGS.

Many studies confirm that sleep loss keeps you hungry, searching for calories in the form of sugary snacks and starches. Bottom line: Inadequate sleep can cause you to put on pounds.

IT MAY TRIGGER A PERSONAL ENERGY CRISIS.

All it takes is 6 days of sleep restriction to cause people to develop resistance to insulin, the hormone that helps transport glucose from the bloodstream to the cells, according to University of Chicago researchers. Glucose is the fuel that every cell in your body needs to function properly. If you can't metabolize sugar properly, blood sugar rises, you develop a resistance to insulin, and type 2 diabetes may be in your near future.

IT CAN START A VICIOUS CYCLE.

Inadequate shut-eye causes levels of the stress hormone cortisol to spike late in the day. That triggers increased heart rate, blood pressure, and blood glucose—all the things you don't want to happen when you are preparing for sleep. Guess what? You'll have trouble falling asleep, which triggers more stress hormone, which makes sleep more difficult, which releases more cortisol, which . . . You get the picture of this cyclical nightmare.

the American Sleep Apnea Association. Other options are surgery or sleeping with a CPAP (Continuous Positive Airway Pressure) device, a machine that keeps the airway open with a stream of pressured air. Whatever the treatment, the goal is the same—more restful, uninterrupted sleep. As with any sleep disorder, apnea can lead to excessive daytime sleepiness and cause health consequences like obesity, high blood pressure, and cardiovascular disease. If you wake up with headaches in the morning, suffer from daytime drowsiness, and keep your spouse awake because of your loud snoring, go to a sleep lab for a sleep apnea test. If you're not getting good quality sleep for whatever reason, get to the bottom of it. Your busy body deserves the most restorative rest it can get.

chapter 7

THE GET-BACK-IN-SHAPE WORKOUT

No Matter What Your Level of Fitness, This Plan Will Change Your Life

HERE COULD BE ANY NUMBER of reasons why you suddenly decided that you want to get back into shape. Perhaps you signed up to coach your daughter's soccer team or manage your son's Little League team. Or perhaps you felt a tightness in your hamstring reaching down to tie your shoes and realized—smartly—that this was your body's first warning signal for a bit of needed change. Or maybe, like Joe Maroon, MD, you were performing brain surgery one day, and fueling 18-wheel tractor-trailers and flipping hamburgers at a truck stop in Wheeling, West Virginia, the next.

Dr. Maroon was in his early 40s, with a promising career as a professor of neurological surgery. He had spent his entire life striving to do everything better and faster than everyone else. And he had succeeded. But his preoccupation with career and success began taking its toll on his health and his family. Then disaster struck: Within one week, he lost his father to a heart ➡

attack and his wife and family to a divorce. He was forced to temporarily abandon his surgical practice and his teaching to help his mother run the family business—a truck stop.

"I sank into a pathological depression," says Maroon. "It was the lowest point in my life. Then I picked up an old book I had gotten for high school graduation: *I Dare You!* by William Danforth, the founder of the Ralston Purina Company." In the book, Danforth challenges the reader to lead a life of balance, represented by a box with four equal sides.

"Danforth's instructions called for drawing a square and labeling the sides with the four major components of our life: 'work,' 'family/social,' 'physical,' and 'spiritual,'" says Maroon. "But when I plotted my life, it wasn't a square—it was a flat-line EKG. I saw that my weight gain, depression, and emotional distress were due to the lopsided imbalance in me. . . . My work had become my escape from facing what was going on in my life."

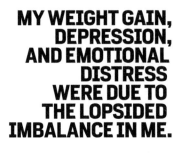

MY WEIGHT GAIN, DEPRESSION, AND EMOTIONAL DISTRESS WERE DUE TO THE LOPSIDED IMBALANCE IN ME.

In his book, *The Longevity Factor*, Maroon describes how that revelation and a return to fitness eventually brought him to a life of balance and health. "I received a phone call from an old friend who asked me to join him for a run. Although I had never enjoyed running, we talked and jogged for four laps around a high school football field, a whole mile, something I hadn't done since college. That evening, for the first time in months, I slept through the night."

The next day Maroon ran a mile and a half, then 2 miles the following day. Eventually, he competed in his first 10K race. While training, the weight started to come off, his mood improved, and his clarity of thought and brain function returned to their former levels. After a year of trying to save his family's business, he was able to return to neurosurgery and repair the spiritual and family/social sides of his life. The balanced-life approach brought new excitement to his medical career, which flourished as a result. For more than 20 years, Maroon has served as team neurosurgeon for the National Football League's Pittsburgh Steelers, and he is currently vice chairman and professor of neurological surgery at the University of Pittsburgh Medical Center as well as a senior vice president of the American Academy of Anti-Aging Medicine. Joe Maroon kept up his exercising, too, adding biking and cycling and, eventually, triathlon competitions. Now 67 (he looks more like 55), he has completed more than 60 triathlons, including the Hawaiian Ironman event (swim 2.4 miles, cycle 112 miles, and run 26.2 miles) and six other Ironman-distance triathlons.

"I've noticed over the years that when one of the four areas—physical, work, family/social, spiritual—is off, I can still function well," he says, "but if two are deficient, my emotional life becomes filled with anxiety and frustration—and I start overeating!" Fortunately, says Maroon, you can regain your balance simply through your deliberate thoughts and actions. "I believe that by consciously focusing on altering the sides of our square, we can actually change our brain anatomy and function."

In what shape is the physical side of your Danforth box? No matter what your reason is for getting back in shape, no matter if you haven't done much more than open the refrigerator door or you are already active and athletic, when you are in your 40s you need to work on three important parts of overall fitness.

➡ FLEXIBILITY Muscles shorten and tighten from lack of use, making you susceptible to injury and triggering symptoms in other parts of the body such as lower back pain. The stretching exercises in Chapter 5 will become your warmup for the workouts that follow.

➡ STRENGTH By doing resistance exercises, you'll raise your metabolism, burn more fat, and prevent age-related muscle loss (sarcopenia). You'll also build power by increasing your fast-twitch muscle fibers and develop a stronger core, which will support your spine and prevent back problems.

➡ **CARDIOVASCULAR CAPACITY** Whether it's through the strength-building circuits or aerobic exercise like walking, running, biking, swimming, and playing sports, you'll improve your lung function and capacity as well as your heart's ability to pump efficiently. Research published recently in the *Journal of Physiology* suggests that vo2 max, one of the best indicators of aerobic fitness, decreases by about 10 percent per decade starting around age 30. (vo2 max, or maximal oxygen uptake, refers to the maximum amount of oxygen that an individual can use during 1 minute of intense exercise. It is measured as milliliters of oxygen used in 1 minute per kilogram of bodyweight.)

But when the researchers at the University of Texas at Austin and the University of Colorado at Boulder tried to find out what causes vo2 max to decline, they were surprised to learn in their study that it was due to reductions in training intensity, not because of any physiological mechanism. What that suggests is that you may be able to maintain your cardiovascular fitness well beyond age 40 through training in specific ways. And this program will help you to do that.

WHAT TO EXPECT:
+THE TOTAL-
BODY PROGRAM

THESE WORKOUTS ARE DESIGNED for people who don't already exercise and want to start, basically, from scratch. We're going to assume you're in the 40-years-and-above demographic or getting pretty near it. That means that we know you have a busy life, a career, maybe a family, and a dozen-and-a-half things tugging at you for your time. So, we've chosen the exercises with all of that in mind.

+ **The workouts are short.** You can do them in 20 to 35 minutes. But they are intense—that's why you can do them in about half an hour! The strength-building moves focus on working the large muscle groups of the chest, back, and legs. That way you'll exercise and build your biggest "landmass," getting the most calorie-burning benefit for your time exercising. Then, we've added a few moves that'll shore up some crucial smaller muscle groups—like those in your shoulders surrounding that vulnerable contraption called the rotator cuff.

+ **You can exercise at home.** Strength Workout #1 is a fast-paced circuit using minimal equipment, so it can be done in your basement, garage, or any small room (just move the ironing board out of the way for safety). You won't have to waste time commuting to a gym or health club to get in a workout if you don't want to. Don't underestimate the time factor. Even a club that's just a mile from your home could be far enough away to convince you to skip a workout. Strength Workout #2 is a more-advanced gym workout, since it includes some exercises that you may not have equipment for at home. However, even this workout features many moves you can do at home with minimal gear. And the aerobic and interval workouts can be done just about anywhere.

+ **You won't need much equipment.** You can get started today by doing the flexibility moves in Chapter 5 and some of the body-weight-only exercises on the following pages. Later, all you'll have to buy are a few simple weights, exercise bands, an exercise bench or step, and a stability ball, also known as a "Swiss ball." We recommend getting a few pairs of dumbbells in varying weights. In your 40s, your joints can become sensitive; using dumbbells, instead of barbells or machines, can help prevent joint stress by allowing for more freedom of movement. When you go to the gym, we suggest you avoid weight-lifting machines for the most part because they force your muscles to move in a single direction that's often nothing like the way your body moves in real life.

Here's what we have planned for you in this well-rounded strength and aerobic program:

STRENGTH WORKOUT #1

A total-body, at-home circuit of 10 strength-building moves that should take you about 20 minutes to complete. Do this twice a week. You'll do the warmup and cooldown stretches found in Chapter 5 before and after each workout.

STRENGTH WORKOUT #2

A total-body gym-based routine that is performed more slowly using heavier resistance. Do this 35-minute workout once a week. You can do these two basic strength workouts for months by increasing the weight as you get stronger and mixing in other exercises to keep your muscles challenged.

CORE WORKOUT

These exercises will shore up your midsection and prevent back problems down the road. No traditional hands-behind-the-head crunches! That's right, this core workout involves no crunches for your abs, but that doesn't mean they'll be a snap. They focus on more important stability muscles than the for-show rectus abdominus! You'll do a core workout 2 days a week, attached to any of the strength or light-cardio workouts.

AEROBIC WORKOUT

Aerobic workouts build cardiovascular fitness. Ours include brisk walking, which is perfect for those who've been sedentary for a long while, plus more-advanced interval training workouts for running, biking, or swimming. You will do an aerobic workout 2 or 3 days a week: 1 day for light cardiovascular exercise such as walking or cycling; 1 day for a high-intensity interval workout; and an optional cross-training/fun day for biking with your family, volleyball, softball, swimming, skating, canoeing, martial arts, yoga—you name it.

EXPLOSIVE, THEN STEADY:
+TWO WAYS TO BUILD STRENGTH

CHOOSE WHICH DAYS OF THE WEEK you'll do your three strength workouts, **Strength Workout #1** twice and **Strength Workout #2** once. You might decide Monday, Wednesday, and Friday, or Tuesday, Thursday, and Saturday, leaving Sunday for rest. It doesn't matter, as long as you leave a day between strength workouts for muscle recovery and repair.

Rest is crucial. It's during those "off" days when your muscles will grow. Here's how it happens: When you do a biceps curl or any resistance-training move, the stress causes tiny tears in your muscle fibers. This muscle breakdown triggers amino acids to come to the rescue, like microscopic EMTs, to patch up the tiny traumas. This repair reinforces muscle fibers, making them stronger and bigger. That's how muscle grows.

All this first-aid requires energy, which explains why your metabolism rises in the hours after a tough workout. A University of Wisconsin study found that when subjects performed a full-body resistance workout involving three big-muscle exercises— the squat, bench press, and power clean—their metabolisms were elevated for 39 hours afterward! That post-workout calorie-frying is what's known as the after-burn effect of exercise.

To keep **Strength Workout #1** short and efficient, we recommend doing two sets of each exercise for 12 to 15 repetitions. "Two sets of fairly heavy weight will give you more than 80 percent of the benefit you'll get from lifting weights, so there's no need to spend hours in a weight room," says Vonda Wright, MD, an orthopedic surgeon and assistant team physician for the University of Pittsburgh Panthers football team. "Even one set of 12 repetitions using at least 65 percent of your one-rep maximum is enough to build and maintain muscle and strength."

➡ **STRENGTH WORKOUT #1** should be done in a circuit-training fashion, twice a week. Circuit training is a common style of organizing a workout in which you perform one exercise, and then move on to a different exercise with very little rest in between, and so on and so on. It's best to pair exercises that focus on opposing muscle groups back-to-back in a circuit. For example, you might do bench presses first, which work the chest muscles, followed by bent-over rows, which work the muscles of the back. In this way, you can trim the rest time between exercises because you don't have to wait for your chest to recover; your back muscles are fresh and ready to go. Working different muscle groups in a quick-moving circuit may shave 10 minutes off your total workout. What's more, working opposing muscles back-to-back ensures that you'll build a more balanced physique.

You've heard of muscle memory? Well, muscles are creatures of habit, and they will quickly fall into a routine if you don't change things every now and again. By doing the same workout over and over again, your muscles will adapt and learn to do them efficiently, which means they won't be as challenged as they were the first time you did the workout. So trainers and exercise physiologists recommend switching exercise order, adding new exercises, or simply altering how much weight you use or how quickly you move it. And we'll do that within these workouts.

For your two circuit-training workouts, we recommend you use resistance (dumbbells, mostly) that amounts to 60 to 80 percent of your one-repetition maximum. In other words, find out how much weight you can bench press once using good form without struggling. Use a weight that's 60 to 80 percent of that number for your 12 to 15 reps. Another way to ballpark your workout weight: Select a weight that's heavy enough to make you struggle to get through the last two reps.

How fast should each rep be done? Quickly. We recommend lowering the weight for 2 seconds, pausing for 1 second, and then lifting the weight explosively. The stress created by this quick, explosive burst builds muscle power, just the kind you need as you travel beyond the age of 40. Remember the research done by Tufts University professor Roger Fielding, which showed that rapid weight-lifting made subjects' muscles more powerful than traditional slow lifting did, because it spurred the growth of fast-twitch muscles. Not only will you lift quickly during these two circuits, you'll incorporate some explosive plyometric moves to keep the spring in your step.

➡ **STRENGTH WORKOUT #2,** your middle strength-training workout of the week, should be done as straight sets—that is, you will complete one set of an exercise, rest for 30 seconds to a minute, then complete the second set before moving on to a different exercise. We recommend you surprise your muscles by using heavier weights and slowing down your reps for this workout. Use 80 percent of the weight you can lift once, and reduce the number of reps to between five and eight, this time. Take 3 seconds on the lowering phase and 2 seconds on the lifting phase. Arizona State University researchers studying lifting techniques found that men who alternated the number of repetitions between workouts gained twice as much strength as those who did the same number every time.

WALK, THEN *MOTOR*:
+LIGHT-CARDIO AND INTERVAL TRAINING

ON THE DAYS BETWEEN YOUR STRENGTH WORKOUTS, do some light cardiovascular exercise. Brisk walking for about 20 minutes is perfect, and it's something even beginners can do. Easy cycling or casual swimming is good, too—something to keep you loose, elevate your heart rate and make you sweat.

As your fitness improves, we recommend doing one light-cardio workout, one intense interval-training workout, and one cross-training exercise or sport that works your muscles in a different manner than walking, running, or road biking does. For the cross-training, you can do biking, lap swimming, tennis, basketball, skating, yoga, tai chi, canoeing, hiking, or trail running. Anything will do that elevates your heart rate and works muscles, but is not too intense.

Interval training is much more intense. Like those strength circuits, it delivers a powerful cardiovascular and aerobic workout in a short period of time. Intervals are short bursts of high-intensity "work" followed by "active rest" periods. Studies show that interval training can help build muscle and accelerate aerobic fitness in about a quarter of the time it would take in traditional slow endurance training. Canadian researchers found that athletes who used interval training burned nine times more fat than athletes who didn't use intervals. What's more, interval training has been shown to raise metabolism and keep it high, mimicking the after-burn effect of weight training.

You can do intervals with running, cycling, swimming, jumping rope; you can do them on a treadmill, stair climber, elliptical trainer, or rowing ergometer. As your fitness improves, gradually increase the time and number of intervals you perform. On the following pages are two very easy walk/run intervals, as well as more-advanced (faster-paced) interval workouts.

Here's one option for your week's workout schedule followed by the details, broken down by day.

MON	TUES	WED	THURS	FRI	SAT	SUN
stretch	stretch	stretch	stretch	stretch	stretch	rest
strength workout #1	aerobic: light cardio	strength workout #2	aerobic: intervals	strength workout #1	aerobic: cross-train (optional)	
	core			core		

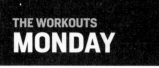
STRENGTH WORKOUT #1

Loosen up with the Warmup Moves and Stretches detailed in Chapter 5. Then do the 10 exercises listed below in two circuits: Complete one set of each exercise in order without resting between exercises, rest 5 minutes (after the first circuit), then repeat the circuit. Cool down with the post-workout stretches listed in "Stretching for Exercise" on page 95.

EXERCISE	REPETITIONS	SETS
Warmup Moves and Stretches		1
Goblet Squat	12-15	2 (one set in each circuit)
High Step-Up	12-15 each leg	2
Step Pushup	10-20	2
Single-Arm Dumbbell Row	12-15 each arm	2
Biceps Curl	12-15	2
Triceps Kickback	12-15 each arm	2
Scaption	12-15	2
Explosive Jump	12-15	2
Internal Shoulder Rotation	12-15 each arm	2
External Shoulder Rotation	12-15 each arm	2
Cooldown Stretches		1 (only after the second circuit)

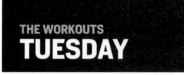

LIGHT-CARDIO AND BASIC CORE WORKOUT

Do a selection of Warmup Moves and Stretches from Chapter 5, then a brisk walk or bike ride for 20 to 30 minutes. Once you improve your aerobic fitness, turn this light walking workout into a run or other moderate–intensity cardio workout. Finish with the Basic Core exercises listed in the chart.

EXERCISE	REPETITIONS	SETS/DURATION	REST
Warmup Moves and Stretches		1	
Brisk walk or bike ride		20 to 30 minutes	

BASIC CORE WORKOUT			
Superman	10	1	15 seconds
Hip Extension	20	1	15 seconds
Arm and Leg Raising and Lowering	20	1	15 seconds
Bird Dog	20	1	15 seconds
Two-Handed Wood Chop	10 on each side	1	15 seconds

STRENGTH WORKOUT #2

Start with your Warmup Moves and Stretches. Complete two sets of each exercise before moving on to the next exercise. For this workout, use a heavier weight than in Strength Workout #1 (except for the Side-Lying External Rotation), a weight heavy enough that your last repetition is very challenging.

EXERCISE	REPETITIONS	SETS	REST
Warmup Moves and Stretches		1	
Barbell Front Squat	5–8	2	30–60 seconds
Dumbbell Forward Lunge	5–8	2	30–60 seconds
Dumbbell Incline Bench Press	5–8	2	30–60 seconds
Seated Cable Row	5–8	2	30–60 seconds
Biceps Curl to Overhead Press	5–8	2	30–60 seconds
Cable Triceps Pressdown	5–8	2	30–60 seconds
Deadlift	5–8	2	30–60 seconds
Front Lat Pulldown	5–8	2	30–60 seconds
Side-Lying External Rotation	10 each arm	2	30–60 seconds
High Knee Skips	20	2	30–60 seconds
Plyometric Box Jumps	10	2	3–5 minutes
Cooldown Stretches		1	

THE WORKOUTS
THURSDAY

20- TO 30-MINUTE CARDIO AND INTERVAL WORKOUT

Start with your Warmup Moves and Stretches. Choose one of the following interval workouts, or make up your own. End with Cooldown Stretches.

EASY
Interval 1
+ 5 minutes walk
+ 15 minutes run/walk

(total: 20 minutes)

Interval 2
+ 5 minutes walk
+ 20 minutes run/walk done faster
+ 5 minutes walk

(total: 30 minutes)

ADVANCED
Interval 3
+ Warm up:
  5 minutes brisk walk
  3 minutes moderate-paced run (to increase heart rate)
+ Work:
  1 minute increased speed (not a sprint, but you're moving)

+ Active rest:
  3 minutes decreased speed to a comfortable pace (to lower heart rate)
+ Work:
  1 minute: increased speed for the first 30 seconds, then 90 percent of maximum speed for the next 30 seconds
+ Active rest:
  3 minutes decreased speed to a comfortable pace
+ Work:
  1 minute: increased speed for the first 30 seconds, then all out for the next 30 seconds
+ Active rest:
  3 minutes decreased speed to a comfortable pace

+ Cool down:
  5 minutes walk, briskly at first, then casually for the last 2 minutes

(total: 25 minutes)

Interval 4
+ Warm up:
  5 minutes slow jog
  4 minutes moderate-paced run
+ Work:
  30 seconds increased speed to 80 percent of your best effort
+ Active rest:
  90 seconds decreased speed to a comfortable pace (alternate between Work and Active Rest phases, six to eight times)
+ Cool down:
  3 minutes slow jog, 2 minutes walk

(total: 26 to 30 minutes)

The Knee-Saving Interval

Try this elliptical machine workout to spare your joints

Weak in the knees? Elliptical machines are perfect to avoid the hammering foot strikes that can transmit hundreds of pounds of force to your knees. University of Mississippi researchers found that exercising on ellipticals delivers the same cardiovascular benefits as running on treadmills, without the jarring impact. But they are just about worthless if you use them incorrectly. Keep your hands off the handles; leaning on them lightens the load on your legs, which cheats you out of a good workout. Instead, pump your arms as if you are running. Another common way people unwittingly sabotage their elliptical workout is by allowing the momentum of the cycling foot pedals to move their feet. Make sure your legs are doing the work. Try this 20- to 30-minute workout, which alternates between high resistance and high speed.

1

3 to 5 minutes of warmup at an easy pace and light resistance

2

2 minutes of high resistance at a slow pace

3

2 minutes of low resistance at a fast pace

4

Repeat the 4-minute sequence three to five times, depending on your level of fitness.

5

3 to 5 minutes of cool down at an easy pace and light resistance

6

Don't forget to stretch your hamstrings, quads, and calves after the workout.

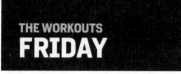

THE WORKOUTS

FRIDAY

STRENGTH WORKOUT #1 AND ADVANCED CORE ROUTINE

Start with the Warmup Moves and Stretches. Complete 1 set of each exercise in order, rest 5 minutes, then repeat the circuit. Rest for a few minutes, then do a core workout. You may repeat the Basic Core routine shown listed on Monday's chart or try the Advanced Core exercises listed below. After the core moves, do a brief cool down.

EXERCISE	REPETITIONS	SETS
Warmup Moves and Stretches		1
Goblet Squat	12-15	2 (one in each circuit)
High Step-Up	12-15 each leg	2
Step Pushup	10-20	2
Single-Arm Dumbbell Row	12-15 each arm	2
Biceps Curl	12-15	2
Triceps Kickback	12-15 each arm	2
Scaption	12-15	2
Explosive Jump	12-15	2
Internal Shoulder Rotation	12-15 each arm	2
External Shoulder Rotation	12-15 each arm	2

ADVANCED CORE WORKOUT		
Leg-Lowering Drill	10-20	rest 15 seconds
Stability Ball Pull-in	10-20	rest 15 seconds
V-Spread Toe Touch	10-20	rest 15 seconds
Side Plank	10-20	rest 15 seconds
Side Plank with Reach Under	10-20 on each side	
Cooldown Stretches		1

Stretching for Exercise

Here's how to warm up and cool down when working out

WARM-UP STRETCHES	DURATION
Prisoner Squat	10-15 reps
Trunk Rotation	10 reps
Knee Hug to Lunge	10 reps with each leg
Inch worm	5 reps
Hip Circle	5 reps with each leg, hold 10 seconds
Inch worm	10 reps with each leg
Butt stretch	30 seconds with each leg
Airplane	5 reps with each leg, hold 10 seconds
Back Lunge and Twist	10 reps with each leg
Butterfly stretch	15-30 seconds
Calf stretch	30 seconds
Anterior shoulder stretch	15 seconds with each arm

COOLDOWN STRETCHES	DURATION
Calf stretch	30 seconds
Hamstring stretch	30 seconds with each leg
Butt stretch	30 seconds with each leg
Quad stretch	30 seconds with each leg
Anterior shoulder stretch	15 seconds with each arm

+THE EXERCISES
STRENGTH WORKOUT#1

GOBLET SQUAT

1 Hold a heavy dumbbell vertically in front of your chest by grasping one end of the weight with both hands. Stand with your feet shoulder width apart.

2 Push your hips backward, then bend your knees and squat as deeply as you can. Keep your back and head as upright as possible throughout the lift.

3 Push yourself quickly back to the starting position.

Do 12 to 15 reps.

➡ **TIP: Full squats like this strengthen knee tendons better than half squats, which tend to overdevelop quadriceps. Perfect the technique before using heavier weights.**

HIGH STEP-UP

1 Stand in front of an exercise bench or a step that's 12 to 18 inches off the ground—high enough to create a 90–degree angle at the knee.

2 Place your left foot on the bench and push your body up until your left leg is straight and you are standing on that one leg on the bench, your right foot hanging behind the bench.

3 Lower your body until your right foot touches the floor. That's one repetition. Then immediately press your left foot into the bench again to lift yourself up. Do 12 to 15 reps, and then repeat the exercise using your right leg.

➡ *TIP:* Focus on pushing down through your heel, rather than your toes. That will help you keep your knee over your ankle. Extending your knee over your toes can lead to injury. Hold a pair of dumbbells to make the exercise more challenging.

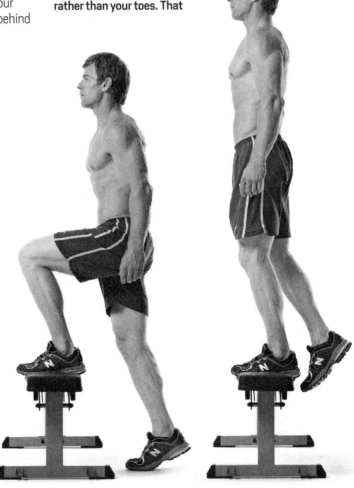

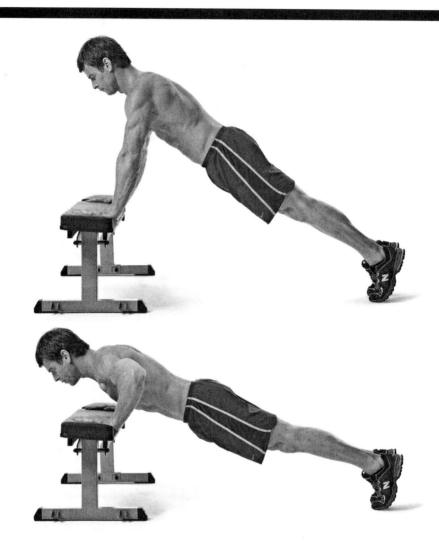

STEP PUSHUP

1 Get into a pushup position, but instead of placing your hands on the floor, place them on a stair-step or other stable structure that's raised a few inches off the floor.
2 With your arms extended straight, keep your back flat and your face down, and contract your abs. Bend your elbows and lower yourself until your chest is an inch off the step. Pause a second, then explosively push yourself up. Do 10 to 20 reps.

➡ **TIP:** This is a great chest move for those who aren't strong enough for regular pushups. The higher the step, the easier it will be to perform the pushup. As you get stronger, progressively lower the elevation. Once you become proficient enough to knock out 20 hands-on-the-floor pushups, try elevated-feet pushups, even harder, in which you rest your toes on the step and place your hands on the floor.

SINGLE-ARM DUMBBELL ROW

1 Grab a dumbbell in your left hand and bend forward, placing your right hand and right knee on a flat bench. Keep your back flat and your upper body parallel to the floor. Let your left arm hang straight down from your shoulder with your palm facing inward.

2 Raise your left upper arm up until it's just past parallel to the floor, with your elbow above the level of your torso. Pause, lower the weight, and repeat. Do 12 to 15 reps, then repeat the exercise with your right hand holding the dumbbell and your left hand and knee on the bench.

➡ *TIP:* For a change of pace, try a Dumbbell Piston Row. You won't need a bench. Stand with legs shoulder-width apart and hold a dumbbell in each hand. (They should be lighter than the ones you use for single-arm rows.) Bend at the waist and allow the weights to hang below you. With your palms facing each other, rapidly row each dumbbell up to the side of your chest in alternating-arm fashion— like a piston.

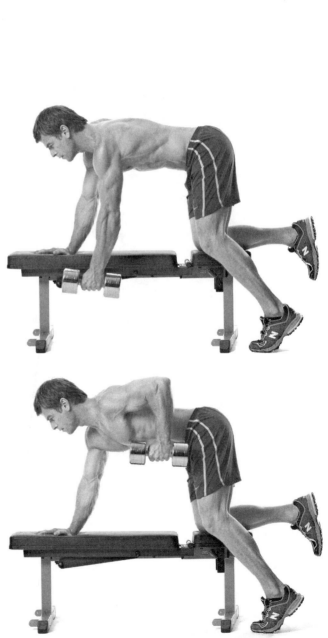

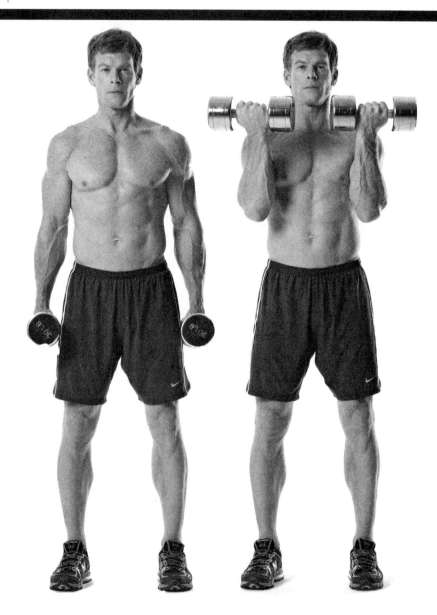

BICEPS CURL

1 Stand with your feet shoulder-width apart and a dumbbell in each hand at your sides, palms facing inward.

2 Keeping your upper arms perfectly still, curl the weights up quickly, rotating to an underhand grip, until they reach the front of your shoulders. Lower the weights more slowly, to a 2-count.

Do 12 to 15 reps.

➡ **TIP:** If your wrists hurt, don't rotate your hands to an underhand grip, but keep your palms facing inward as you curl your arms.

TRICEPS KICKBACK

1 Stand next to a bench holding a lightweight dumbbell in your left hand. Bend forward and place your right knee and right hand on a bench. Your torso should be parallel with the floor and your right leg should be under your hips for support.

2 Bend your right arm and press the inside of your elbow against your side so that your upper arm is parallel with the floor and the dumbbell rests next to your chest, your palm facing inward.

3 Slowly, press the weight back behind you until your arm is straight. Pause a second, then return the weight to your chest by bending your arm but keeping your elbow stationary. Complete 12 to 15 reps, then repeat the exercise with your right arm, placing your left knee and left hand on the bench.

➡ **TIP:** This lift trains the muscles in the backs of your arms, which are susceptible to atrophy. Moving your elbow during the lift is cheating.

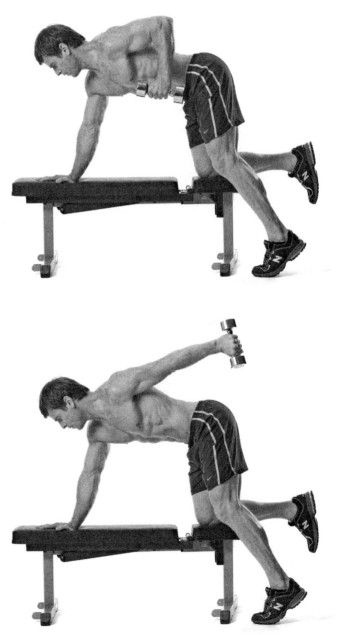

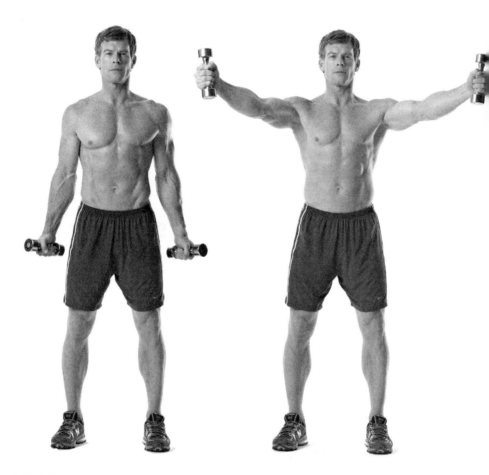

SCAPTION

1 Stand straight with your feet shoulder-width apart. Hold a lightweight dumbbell in your hands at your sides.

2 Rotate the dumbbells so that your thumbs are up (palms facing inward) and raise your arms up to shoulder height at a 45-degree angle from your torso. Your arms should make a Y shape in front of you. As you raise your arms, pull in and depress your scapulas (shoulder blades). Be careful to avoid shrugging your shoulders to raise the weight. Once the dumbbells reach shoulder height, lower them following that same Y-shaped path. Do 12 to 15 reps.

➡ *TIP:* **Perform this exercise in front of a mirror to check your form. This movement, which exercises the supra-spinatus muscle, a part of the rotator cuff, is important for healthy shoulder-joint mechanics.**

EXPLOSIVE JUMP

1 Stand with your feet slightly more than hip–width apart. Swing your arms back as you dip down and bend the hips and knees.

2 Drive your arms forward and up as you jump explosively off the floor. Immediately dip down and repeat.

Do 12 to 15 reps.

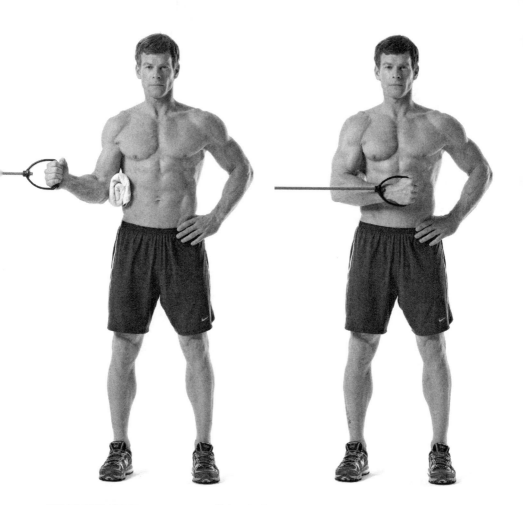

INTERNAL SHOULDER ROTATION WITH BAND

1 Tie a length of exercise tubing or stretch band to a fixed object that's about hip-high at your right side. Hold the other end of the tube or band in your right hand with your elbow bent to 90 degrees, your upper arm and elbow pressed against your side, and your forearm parallel with the floor. For a greater range of motion, add a small rolled towel between your arm and side. The palm of your right hand should face inward. Step to the side away from the fixed object to stretch the band.

2 Keeping your elbow by your side, move your hand toward your stomach as far as is comfortable. Slowly release under tension to return to the starting position. Do 12 to 15 reps. Then turn around and repeat the exercise using your left arm.

➡ *TIP:* **This move and the external rotation that follows are the safest ways to strengthen your shoulder joint.**

EXTERNAL SHOULDER ROTATION WITH BAND

1 Tie a length of exercise tubing or stretch band to a fixed object that's about hip-high and to your left side. Hold the other end of the tube or band in your right hand with your elbow bent to 90 degrees, your upper arm and elbow pressed against your side, and your forearm parallel with the floor. The palm of your right hand should face in toward your torso. Step to the side away from the fixed object to stretch the band. Your forearm should rest, under the tension of the band, against your stomach.

2 Pivoting on your elbow still pressed against your side, move your right forearm out and away from you as far as is comfortable. Pause a second, then slowly release, bringing your hand back across your body. Do 12 to 15 reps, then switch sides and perform the exercise using your left arm.

➡ *TIP:* Use a rolled towel to make the exercise more effective.

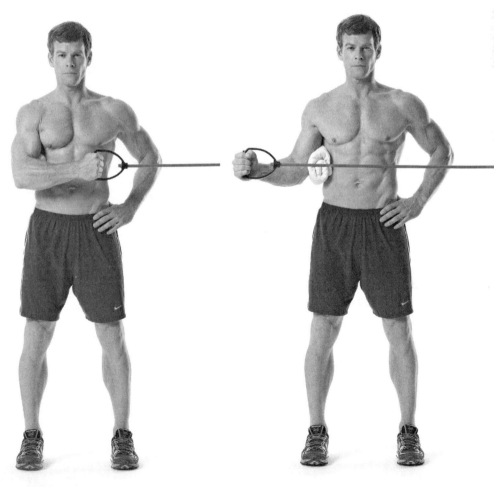

+THE EXERCISES
STRENGTH WORKOUT#2

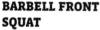

BARBELL FRONT SQUAT

1 Grab a barbell with an overhand grip, your hands just beyond shoulder width on the bar. Lift it up and hold it against the front of your body, just above your shoulders. Raise your upper arms so they are just about parallel to the floor, allowing the bar to roll back against your shoulders and on top of your fingers. Place your feet shoulder–width apart, and keep your knees slightly bent, your back straight, and eyes forward.

2 Slowly lower your body by bending your knees as if sitting into a chair, keeping your back in its natural alignment. When your thighs are a bit lower than parallel to the floor, pause, then push forcefully with your legs to return to the starting position. Do 5 to 8 reps.

➡ **TIP:** You can squat as low as you can comfortably go; the lower you go, the better the stress on your muscles. This classic exercise is important for hip, trunk, and leg strength and postural stability.

DUMBBELL FORWARD LUNGE

1 Stand with your feet together, holding a dumbbell in each hand at your sides, palms facing in.

2 Take a large step forward with your left leg. When your front thigh is parallel to the floor and your back knee is a few inches off the floor, hold for 1 second. Then return to the starting position, and repeat with your right leg. Do 5 to 8 reps.

➡ *TIP:* Be sure to keep your knee from extending over your toes, which can cause injury. Lunges can be done without weights if you find the exercise too difficult using dumbbells.

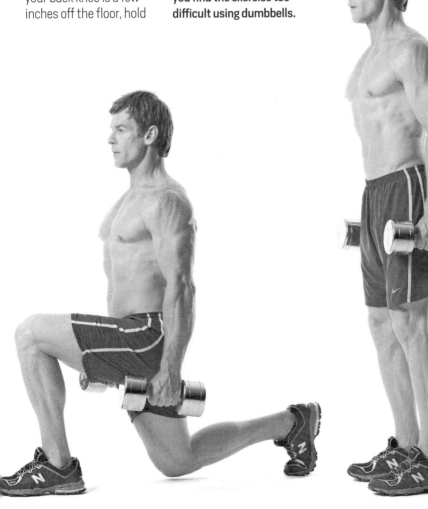

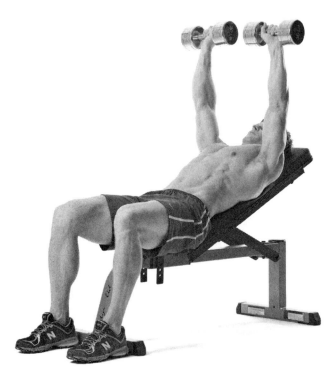

DUMBBELL INCLINE BENCH PRESS

1 Lie on an incline bench with feet flat on the floor. Hold a pair of dumbbells above your chest, arms extended, using an overhand grip.

2 Lower the dumbbells toward the sides of your chest (stop when your elbows are at torso level or just a little lower), pause, and then quickly push them back up to the starting position. Do 5 to 8 reps.

➡ *TIP:* The bench should not be tilted more than 30 degrees for this lift.

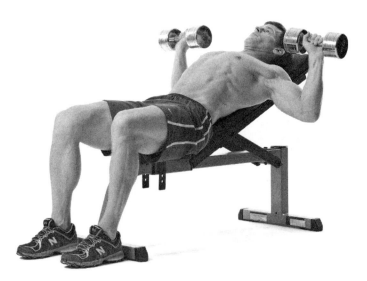

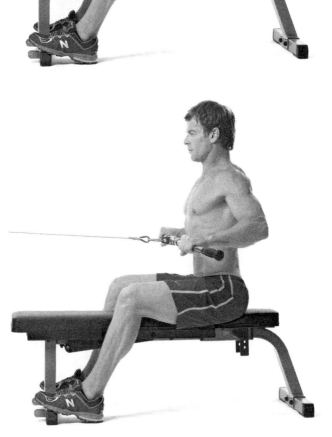

SEATED CABLE ROW

1 Sit at a cable row station, or attach a straight bar to a cable machine. Grasp the handle with both hands using an overhand grip. Sit up with a straight back, brace your feet, and pull your shoulders back.

2 Forcefully pull the bar to your abdomen by bending your arms and squeezing your shoulder blades together. Pause for a second with your blades together, then take 2 seconds to return to the starting position. Don't lean forward on the return. Do 5 to 8 reps.

➡ **TIP:** For best results, make sure your hands are about shoulder-width apart on the bar and that you don't bend forward and backward at the waist.

BICEPS CURL TO OVERHEAD PRESS

1 Stand with your feet shoulder-width apart and a dumbbell in each hand at your sides, palms facing forward.

2 Curl both arms upward while turning the backs of your hands outward to an underhand grip.

3 When the dumbbells reach your shoulders, press them overhead while twisting your hands inward so that your palms face forward at the top of the lift. Do 5 to 8 reps.

➡ **TIP: If you have rotator cuff impingement, avoid the overhead press part of this lift.**

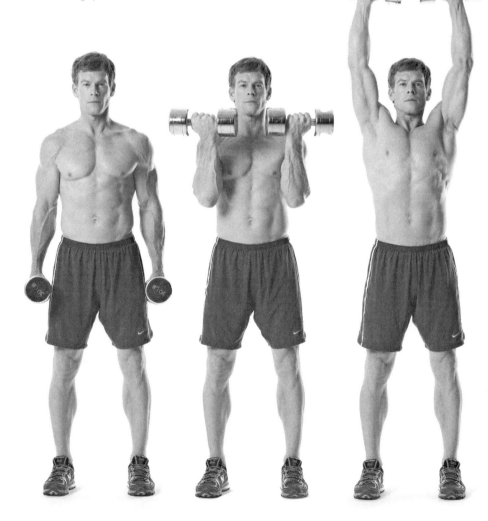

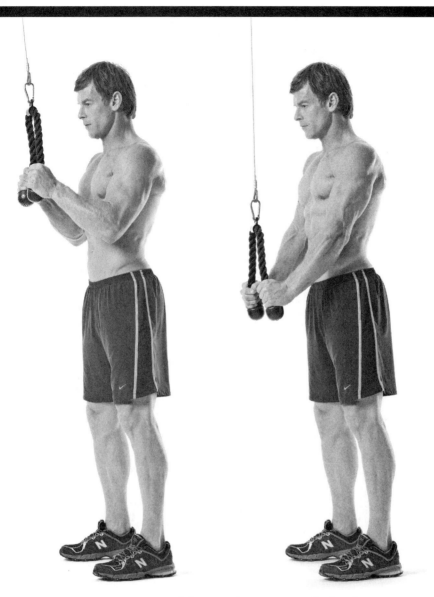

CABLE TRICEPS PRESSDOWN

1 Attach a rope or V-bar to an overhead cable pulley station. Stand facing the station with your feet shoulder-width apart. Grasp the rope, palms facing inward, and pull down until your arms are bent at about a 90-degree angle.

2 Keeping your upper arms close to your body and your elbows from moving, push down on the rope until your arms are almost straight.

Do 5 to 8 reps.

➡ **TIP:** Avoid using your shoulders to cheat the weight down by concentration on keeping your elbows locked against your sides. You won't need a lot of weight if you do this correctly.

211

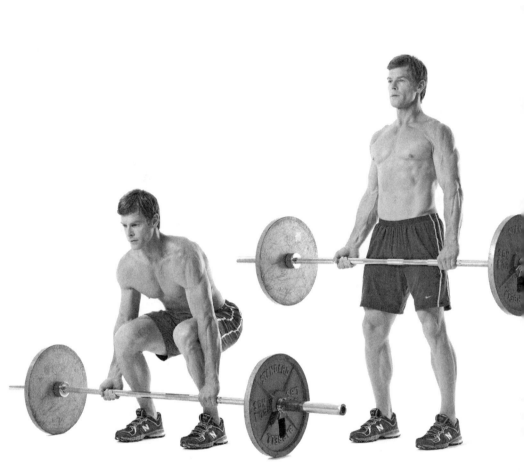

DEADLIFT

1 Stand with the bar on the floor in front of you so it just touches your shins.

2 Push your hips back and grasp the bar with your hands just outside of your calves, one hand using an overhand grip, the other grabbing the bar underhand.

3 Keeping your back straight and chest up, forcefully drive your heels into the floor, and stand up.

4 Then lower the bar back to the floor. Do 5 to 8 reps.

➡ **TIP:** To improve your form, imagine a string attached to your head, pulling you up like a puppet. This will keep you from hunching and hitching.

FRONT LAT PULLDOWN

1 Stand facing a lat pulldown machine. Reach up and grasp the bar with an overhand grip that's 4 to 6 inches wider than your shoulders. Sit on the seat, letting the resistance of the bar extend your arms above your head.

2 Pull the bar down until it touches your upper chest. Hold this position for a second, then return to the starting position. Do 5 to 8 reps.

➡ *TIP:* To avoid injury, don't bring the bar down behind your head.

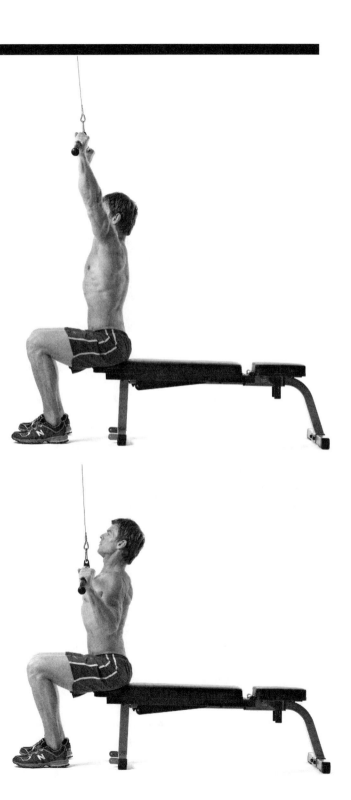

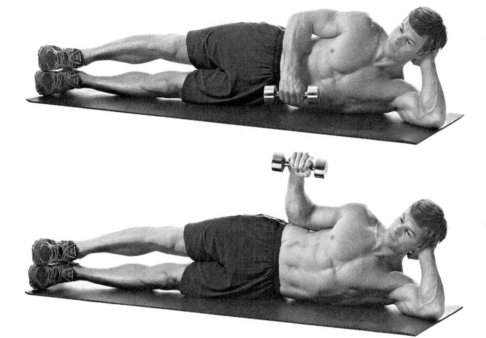

SIDE-LYING SINGLE ARM EXTERNAL ROTATION

1 Lie on your left side with your left arm bent and your head resting on your left hand. Hold a light dumbbell in your right hand. Important: It should be only 1 to 2 pounds; you don't want to use anything much heavier for the delicate rotator cuff. Bend your right arm 90 degrees and tuck your upper arm against your right side. Let the weight hang in front of your midsection.

2 Keeping your upper arm stationary, slowly rotate your forearm until it points toward the ceiling. Then rotate your forearm back to the starting position. Do 10 reps. Then turn over and repeat the exercise with your left arm.

➡ **TIP: If you don't have 1- or 2-pound dumbbells, use a large soup can for resistance. You'll risk injury with anything much heavier.**

HIGH KNEE SKIPS

1 Keeping your upper body straight, drive a knee as high up and out as you can, alternating your knees while skipping. As you drive each knee up, swing your opposite hand up to get as much vertical lift as possible. Do about 20 skips.

➡ *TIP:* For a smoother rhythm, add a hop on the downward step.

PLYOMETRIC BOX JUMPS

1 Stand in front of a stable box or step that's 12 to 18 inches high. Crouch down while throwing your arms behind you. Then swing your arms forward as you explosively jump onto the box.

2 Land on both feet, stand, then lightly jump forward off the box, landing in a crouch to absorb the impact. Turn around to face the box again. Do 10 reps.

➡ *TIP:* **This power move works your entire lower body, especially your hamstrings and gluteals.**

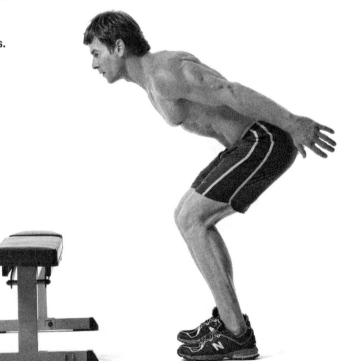

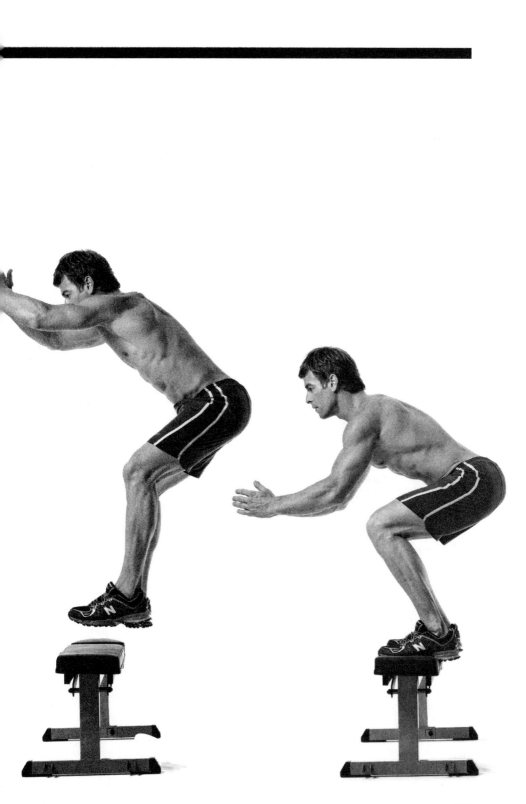

+CORE EXERCISES
BASIC CORE WORKOUT

SUPERMAN

1 Lie face down with your arms extended straight out in front of your head, palms on the floor.

2 Extend your back, lifting your arms, head, and chest while also lifting your legs. Hold that position for 2 seconds, then return to the starting position. Do 10 reps.

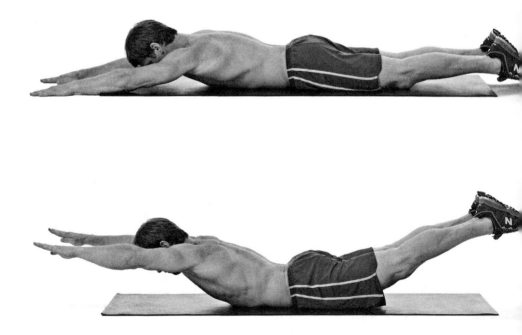

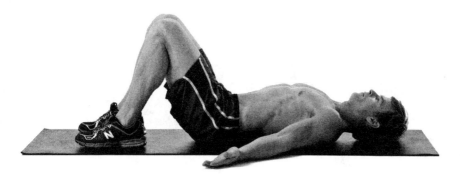

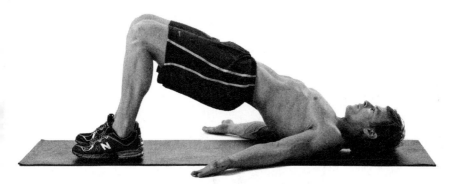

HIP EXTENSION

1 Lie on your back on the floor with your knees bent to 90 degrees and your feet flat on the floor. Place your arms at your sides with your hands palms up and a few inches away from your hips.

2 Raise your hips so your body forms a straight line from your shoulders to your knees. Hold for 2 seconds while tightening your abdominals and buttocks.

3 Take 2 seconds to lower yourself to the starting position. Do 20 reps.

➡ **TIP:** You can make this exercise more difficult by doing the hip–thigh extension. From the starting position, extend your left leg out straight on the floor. Now, as you raise your hips, raise that straight leg until that leg forms a straight line from your foot to your shoulders. Complete the repetitions, then do the exercise with your right leg extended.

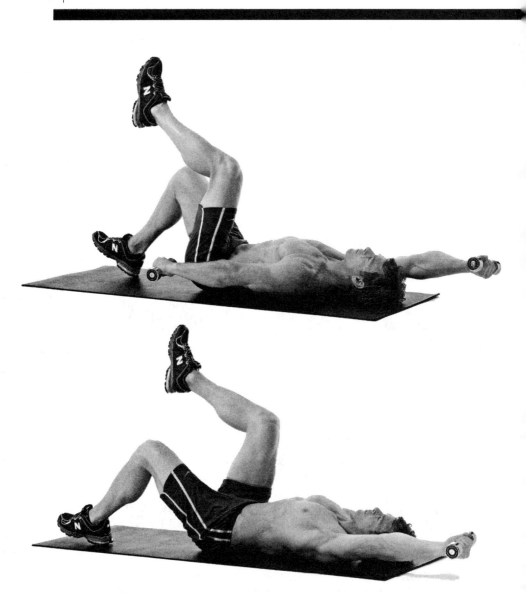

ARM AND LEG RAISING AND LOWERING

1 Grab two light-weight dumbbells and lie on the floor with your knees bent, feet on the floor, and your arms at your sides. While contracting your abs muscles, lift your right arm over your head while lifting your left bent leg off the floor.

2 Now, lift your left arm (with dumbbell) and right leg while simultaneously lowering your left leg to the floor and your right arm to your side. Continue alternating arm and legs this way: When one arm and leg come up the other arm and leg go down. Do 20 reps.

➡ *TIP:* Try without weights first to get the feel for the movement.

BIRD DOG

1 Get down on all fours with your hands and feet about shoulder-width apart, your back straight, and head in alignment with your back.
2 Lift your left leg out straight behind you while simultaneously lifting your right arm straight out in front of you. Hold for 2 seconds, then switch lifting your right leg out behind you and your left arm out in front. Continue alternating this way. Do 20 reps.

➡ *TIP:* Keep your abs and back tight throughout the movement. This is a good move for people who suffer from low-back pain or would like to firm up their butts.

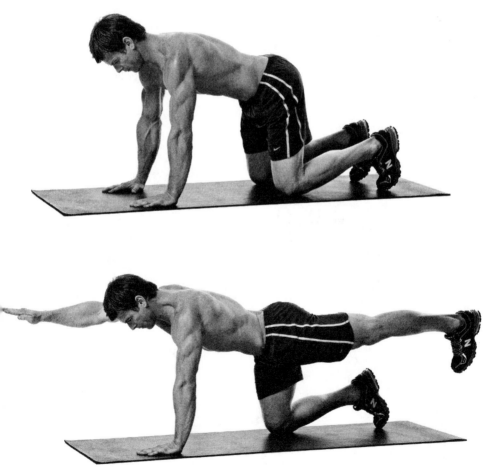

TWO-HANDED WOOD CHOP

1 Stand with your feet shoulder–width apart and your hands holding a light dumbbell above your left shoulder.

2 Rotate your torso to the left as you extend your arms and lower the dumbbell to the outside of your right knee, bending slightly at the waist and knees. Do 10 reps. Then, switch sides, starting with the dumbbell above your right shoulder and moving it toward the outside of your left knee.

➡ **TIP:** Perform this move slowly and under control to avoid allowing the momentum of the dumbbell to wrench your back.

+CORE EXERCISES
ADVANCED CORE WORKOUT

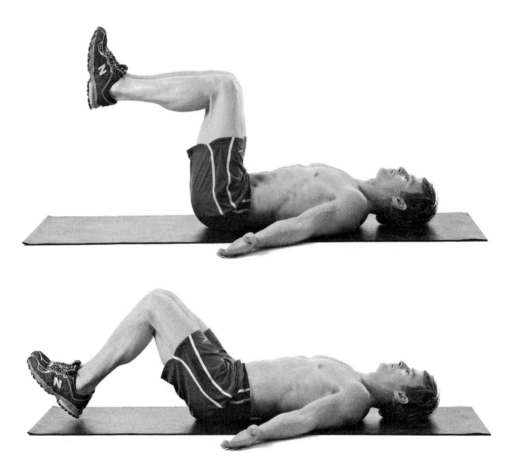

LEG-LOWERING DRILL
1 Lie on your back and raise your legs over your hips, with your knees bent at 90 degrees. Press the small of your back into the floor to eliminate the arch in your lower back.
2 Keep this position as you slowly lower your legs, taking 3 to 5 seconds. Upon reaching the lowest point at which you can still keep your back flat (don't touch your heels to the floor), raise your legs to your chest. Do 10 to 20 reps.
➡ ***TIP:*** Try to lower your **legs farther with each repetition.**

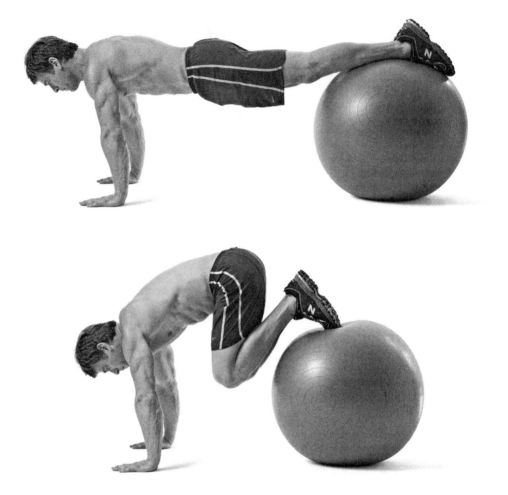

STABILITY BALL PULL-IN

1 Get into a pushup position with your hands slightly more than shoulder-width apart. Instead of placing your feet on the floor, rest your shins on a stability ball. Keep your back flat as you balance.

2 Now, keeping your abs tight and your arms straight, draw your knees toward your chest, rolling the ball toward you until your toes are on top of the ball and your thighs are perpendicular to the ground.

3 Slowly straighten your legs so that the ball rolls back to the starting position. Do 10 to 20 reps.

V-SPREAD TOE TOUCH

1 Lie flat on your back with your legs straight up. Spread your legs slightly to form a V. Raise your arms toward the ceiling between your legs.

2 Curl your shoulder blades up, and reach toward your right foot with both hands while tightening your abs. Hold for a second, then relax back down to the starting position.

3 Next, curl and point toward your left foot and return. Do 10 to 30 reps.

➡ *TIP:* Once you master this move, make it harder by doing it while squeezing a stability ball between your ankles. Hold a light medicine ball in your hands above your head while lying flat with your head on the floor. With arms straight, curl up with the ball in your straight arms, reaching between your legs.

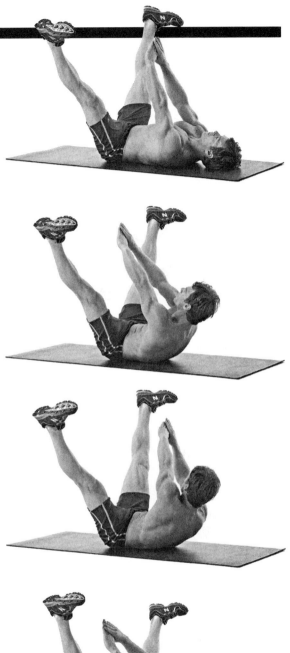

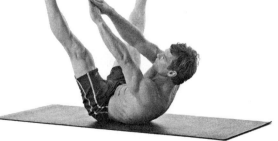

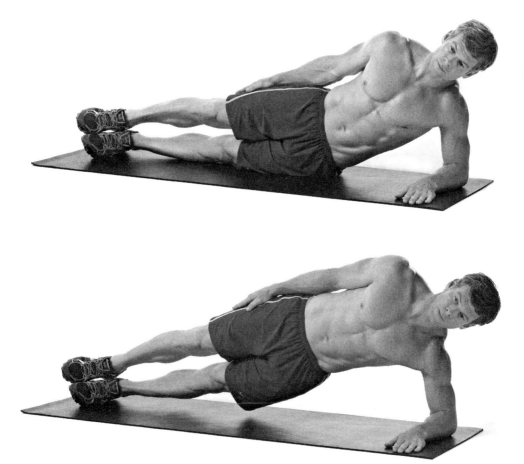

SIDE PLANK

1 Lie on your left side with your knees straight and your feet stacked. Prop your upper body up on your left elbow and forearm, keeping your upper arm directly below your left shoulder.

2 Now, contract your core muscles and raise your hips off the ground so that your body forms a straight line from your ankles to your shoulders. Hold the side plank for 5 seconds, then relax back down and rest for 5 seconds. Do 10 reps. Then repeat the exercise while lying on your right side.

➡ *TIP:* Work up to holding a side plank for 15 to 45 seconds, then repeat the exercise on your right side. Make this exercise more challenging by trying the Side Plank with Reach Under on opposite page.

SIDE PLANK WITH REACH UNDER

1 Lie on your right side with your knees straight and your feet stacked. Prop your upper body up on your left elbow and forearm, keeping your upper arm directly below your left shoulder. Raise your hips off the ground so that your body forms a straight line from your ankles to your shoulders. Lift your right arm and point toward the ceiling with your hand. Hold that position for 2 seconds.

2 While holding that plank, reach under your body with your right hand, then raise it toward the ceiling again. That's one repetition. Do 10 to 20 reps, then lie on your left side and repeat the exercise with your right arm.

➡ *TIP:* **Remember to contract your abs and butt muscles as you are doing the reach move.**

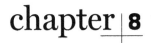

chapter 8

YOUR BODY–
A TROUBLE-SHOOTER'S GUIDE

Regular Health Checks and Quick Fixes That Will Keep You in the Game

OR THE FIRST 30 OR SO YEARS, your body hums along pretty nicely. Sure, there's a glitch and a hiccup here and there—a stretched tendon, a pulled muscle, even a broken bone—but you heal quickly and move on. And most of us sneak through these years relatively unscathed. But your body is a complicated machine, and sometime around your 40s, the machinery requires a bit more attention—call it maintenance. That's when it pays to know a bit about what's going on under the hood, because you don't want to rely on a doctor to tell you everything you need to know to stay healthy. For the record, the average time physicians spend seeing patients is 3 minutes. One hundred eighty seconds. Heck, it takes longer to have your car serviced at Jiffy Lube.

So, Mr. 40+, you need to take charge. And that's what this chapter is about—knowing your body better so you can keep up with the routine maintenance and troubleshoot the sputters ➡

and coughs and aches and pains. Know your body's quirks, and the only thing standing between you and feeling 10 years younger is the right tool for the job.

40,000-Mile Checkup

A good offense, as the saying goes, is the best defense. So, to avoid medical problems, schedule regular physical exams. Guys tend to adopt the "if it ain't broke, don't fix it" mentality toward health care, generally going to see a doctor only when something's wrong. We think this chapter will change your mind.

If your doctor is on the ball, he or she should have given you a major baseline physical exam around age 30. If you haven't had one yet, ask for it. It should include routine stuff such as a head-to-toe physical exam, blood pressure check, hearing and vision tests, a neurological exam, urinalysis, pulmonary-function test, skin cancer check, throat check, and a review of your family health history. But it should also involve more advanced screens such as a complete blood count, body-fat test, bone-density screen, chest x-ray, stress test, kidney and liver function tests, and thyroid function test.

That's a solid baseline checkup for the 30-year-old and a general guideline for future checkups. You should add a baseline EKG to check for heart rhythm abnormalities—and to add to your doctor's file. Do this in your early 40s if you haven't done so already. Now, do yourself a favor and ask your doctor's office to pre-schedule you for annual physicals near your birthday. Each passing year's celebration of your birth is a reminder to give yourself the best birthday present of all—a clean bill of health.

Tests That Can Save Your Life

An at-a-glance guide to checks and screens you should have, and when

WHO	WHAT	WHEN
Everyone	Physical exam	Every 1 to 2 years
	Blood pressure	At least every 2 years
	Lipid panel	At least every 5 years; we recommend yearly
	Diabetes screening	Every 3 years, or as advised
	Vision and glaucoma checkup	Every 2 to 3 years
	Dental checkup	Every year
Everyone at age 50, or earlier if you have a personal history of chronic inflammatory bowel disease or a strong family history of colorectal cancer or polyps	Colonoscopy	Every 10 years, or more if there is a family history of colorectal cancer
	Fecal Occult Blood Test (Stool blood test) *Test can be done at home and samples sent to lab for testing.*	Every year
Everyone starting at age 20	Testicular self-exam	Monthly
Everyone starting at age 50, or earlier if you have a strong family history of prostate cancer or are African American	Discussion with physician about benefits and limitations of the two prostate cancer early-detection tests, the DRE (Digital Rectal Examination) and the PSA (Prostate-Specific Antigen) blood test*	Every year ** See explanation of DRE and PSA on page 234 under "What are the Key Medical Tests All About?"*

+WHAT ARE THE KEY MEDICAL TESTS ALL ABOUT?

CBC, DRE, CRP, FOBT, HDL2. . . .
Wasn't life so much simpler in your 20s when all you had to worry about was avoiding an STD? You've been aware of the tests for sexually transmitted diseases ever since that wild spring break in Cabo. To help you decipher this new medical nomenclature, here's a crib sheet of important tests that anyone over 40 should study. This is good information to get down, because it can help you understand that yellow receipt your doctor's receptionist gives you after you pay the bill. In addition, if your doctor isn't giving you these tests, you can get his attention by saying,

"Hey, doc, how are my homocysteine levels doing?"

BLOOD PRESSURE
A reading of 120/80 mm Hg used to be terrific. Now doctors say that's the low end of "prehypertension" (120/80 to 139/89 mm Hg), which means you're likely to develop high blood pressure if you don't start taking preventive action now. Anything over 140/90 mm Hg is cause for major concern, and medication.

CAROTID DUPLEX ULTRASOUND
Strokes are the third leading cause of death in the United States, and this noninvasive

20-minute test could show if you're at risk. If you're familiar with a pregnancy ultrasound test, the device isn't much different. The technician puts some gel on your neck and then rolls a handheld device over your skin that sends high-frequency sound waves to the carotid arteries. Simple.

The pressure may cause a little mild discomfort, but the exam isn't painful. It provides two views of the arteries in your neck, which reveal damage from plaque buildup and shows how that damage is affecting blood flow to your brain.

Your doctor probably wouldn't order this test unless you have had a stroke or transient ischemic attack (TIA) or she hears an abnormal sound called a bruit through a stethoscope placed over the neck arteries. Still, if you have a family history of stroke or symptoms of heart disease, you may want to consider this test. Eighty percent of all strokes are due to blood clots caused by plaque, and half the time your first symptom is your last. This test isn't normally covered by insurance, but you can get it for just $50 at a handful of private companies.

CBC (COMPLETE BLOOD COUNT)

You must have heard the TV doctors order this one for years. Now you will know what it stands for. Your doctor will likely ask for a CBC if you are complaining of muscle weakness or fatigue so he can check for anemia, infections, or other disorders. But even if you don't have symptoms, it's a good idea to get a baseline record of this array of blood numbers that speak volumes about your overall health. These are the major measures of the CBC test.

➥ **WHITE BLOOD CELL COUNT.** Your white blood cells are your body's department of defense. If you get an infection, the white blood cells spring into action to destroy the virus or bacteria that's infiltrated your airspace. A high white-blood-cell count helps your doctor determine if you have an infection.

➥ **RED BLOOD CELL COUNT.** It's the job of your red blood cells to transport oxygen from the lungs throughout your body and shuttle carbon dioxide back to the lungs so it can be exhaled. A low count is the typical sign of anemia, the most common blood condition in the United States. It suggests that your organs may not be getting the oxygen they need to function.

➡ **HEMATOCRIT AND HEMOGLOBIN COUNTS.** The hematocrit score describes the proportion of red blood cells in your total blood volume. Hemoglobin is the molecule that gives the red blood cell its red color and is responsible for carrying oxygen; its score measures how efficient your blood is at carrying oxygen throughout your body.

➡ **PLATELET COUNT.** Your platelets are the runts of the blood cell litter. Though tiny, they play a huge role in keeping you alive when you receive a paper cut or a gunshot wound. When bleeding happens, the platelets clump together to plug the leak. Too few platelets are a problem, but so are too many. An overabundance can cause hardening of the arteries (atherosclerosis) or form a blood clot in a blood vessel, triggering a heart attack.

CMP (COMPREHENSIVE METABOLIC PANEL)

What sounds like a congressional subcommittee is made up of two blood tests that check for type-2 diabetes. The standard measure is the fasting glucose test. It's often paired with the A1C test, which tracks your average blood-glucose level over several months.

Score high on either one, and your doctor should order an oral glucose tolerance test (OGTT). This one requires about 4 hours and multiple donations of your blood. After taking a blood sample to get a baseline fasting blood glucose level, you'll be given a very sweet liquid to drink. Then, at intervals of 1, 2, and 3 hours, you'll get stuck again. The blood samples measure how efficiently the body's insulin performs its work on the sugar.

COLONOSCOPY

There's good reason to catch colon cancer early: The survival rate is 93 percent if the cancer is treated before it spreads beyond the colon's walls. Of all the tests used to screen for colon cancer, the colonoscopy is the gold standard. The problem with most other tests is that either they don't examine the colon directly (the fecal occult blood test, for example, analyzes your stool for blood) or they don't reach far enough inside your colon. It's a big organ, and half of all colon cancers occur in the half that's not examined by a sigmoidoscopy.

A colonoscopy, however, examines every inch, right up to the small intestine. You should have your first colonoscopy by age 50. If you have a history of colorectal cancer in your family, schedule this test about 10 years earlier than the age of your relative when he was first diagnosed, or in your early 40s.

DEXA SCAN

This test (dual energy x-ray absorpitometry) evaluates bone mineral density to determine the strength of your bones and risk of osteoporosis. You lie on a padded platform for a few minutes while an imaging device passes over your body. Ask your doctor about it if you have two or more osteoporosis risk factors, such as smoking, a family history, excessive alcohol or caffeine use, or a diet low in bone-strengthening calcium.

ENDOTHELIAL FUNCTION ANALYSIS

Your endothelium is the thin membrane that lines the inside of your heart and blood vessels. Studies have shown that endothelial dysfunction is an early warning sign for hardening of the arteries. Now there is a new noninvasive finger test that analyzes the endothelium and is highly predictive of a major cardiac event for people who are considered at low or moderate risk of heart disease.

Called EndoPAT, the device is composed of two probes that look like two large thimbles that are placed on each index finger and hooked up to a small machine that measures blood flow. A blood-pressure cuff is also used. The 15-minute test measures the responsiveness of the endothelial membrane to increased blood flow (physical stress).

In a study conducted by researchers at the Mayo

A New Generation of Cardiac Tests

If you don't score well on your lipid panel, or if you have risk factors for heart disease, ask your doctor to order the new, advanced blood tests that measure small, dense lipoprotein; lipoprotein(a); C-reactive protein; and homocysteine. These are just a few of the advanced metabolic markers that appear on reports from the Berkeley HeartLab, a cardiovascular diagnostics center in San Mateo, California, headed by Robert Superko, MD, author of *Before The Heart Attacks.* These blood tests, and the 64-slice CT scan, represent the cutting edge of heart-disease prevention.

SMALL LDL

The regular cholesterol test measures the amount of LDL cholesterol in your blood, but recently doctors have learned that knowing the particular style of LDL you have makes a big difference. People with a high number of very small, dense forms of LDL cholesterol carry a higher risk of heart attack. People with high, small LDL, also called LDL pattern B, are three times more likely to have coronary artery disease even if their standard cholesterol profile is

Clinic and Tufts-New England Medical Center, 270 patients between ages 42 and 66 who knew they had low-to-medium risk of heart disease were monitored using the device from August 1999 to August 2007. Forty-nine percent of those whose EndoPAT test showed poor endothelial function had a major cardiac event during the 7-year trial.

FASTING LIPID PROFILE

This series of blood tests measures the four components of blood cholesterol. When your blood-test results fall within guidelines deter-

normal and they aren't overweight. This is why some seemingly healthy, thin people with "good" cholesterol numbers surprise us when they suffer heart attacks.

LIPOPROTEIN(A)
High levels of this particle manufactured in your liver also raise your risk of coronary artery disease by as much as 300 percent. Although no lifestyle changes or statin drugs effectively lower Lp(a), having a high score will encourage your doctor to aggressively treat your other metabolic problems.

HOMOCYSTEINE
Homocysteine is an abrasive amino acid that irritates the lining of arteries, opening them up to infiltration by LDL, and may encourage plaque and blood clotting. One study showed that high homocysteine led to an increased risk of stroke, similar to what you get from smoking a pack of cigarettes every day. And it elevates your chances of heart disease by as much as 300 percent!

C-REACTIVE PROTEIN (CRP)
This protein, which is released into the bloodstream, is a tell-tale sign of inflamed arteries. It's twice as effective at predicting heart attacks as LDL. A highly sensitive test (in fact, it's often called high-sensitivity CRP or hs-CRP), it's best to average two scores taken a month apart. If your score is above 3 milligrams per liter, you double your risk of heart attack. And like small LDL, you may have normal cholesterol numbers yet still be at high risk for heart attack with a high CRP score.

64-SLICE CT EXAM
The 64-slice CT (for computed tomography) scan is able to record images so fast that it captures your heart between beats and renders it in 3-D, providing a clearer picture of your coronary arteries than any other type of scan. It detects hard and soft plaques in arteries and gives you a calcium score to gauge your risk of having a heart attack in the future.

mined by the American Heart Association, your doctor will probably conclude that you have nothing to worry about. Conversely, when your numbers are outside of these guidelines, he will recommend lifestyle changes and maybe even cholesterol-lowering drugs.

➡ **TOTAL CHOLESTEROL BELOW 200 MILLIGRAMS PER DECILITER (MG/DL).** This is the weakest value to use to judge the health of your heart. Case in point: In a study of 360,000 men, researchers found that 24 percent of those who died of heart attacks had total cholesterol levels below 200 mg/dL, which is considered healthy.

➡ **HDL ABOVE 45 MG/DL (OPTIMAL IS 60 MG/DL OR HIGHER).** High density lipoprotein (HDL) is called the good cholesterol because high levels seem to protect against heart attack. Theoretically, HDL helps carry bad cholesterol away from the arteries and back to the liver, where it is removed from the body. We do know that low levels correspond with increased heart disease risk. According to data from the Framingham Heart Study, which has been tracking thousands of people since 1948, the average HDL level of men with coronary artery disease is 43.

➡ **LDL BELOW 130 MG/DL (OPTIMAL IS LESS THAN 100 MG/DL, OR LESS THAN 70 MG/DL FOR PEOPLE AT HIGH RISK FOR HEART DISEASE).** This is known as bad cholesterol. Data from Framingham show that the average Low Density Lipoprotein (LDL) cholesterol of those who had heart attacks was 150. The guidelines call that only a "borderline high" risk. If you're at high risk, ask your physician about expanded lipid profile tests. See "A New Generation of Cardiac Tests" on page 238.

➡ **TRIGLYCERIDES BELOW 150 MG/DL.** Triglycerides are a kind of fat in your blood that your body uses for energy. When you have too much, however, you increase your risk for metabolic syndrome, a combination of poor-health factors including high blood sugar, high blood pressure, abdominal fat, and low HDL. Triglyceride levels rise when you eat more calories than you burn, eat a lot of trans fats (mostly from baked goods and chips), and drink a lot of alcohol. You can lower your triglycerides through exercise and by cutting back on high-carb foods like starches, breads, pasta, cookies and cakes, and alcohol.

GLAUCOMA TEST (TONOMETRY)

Nearly a million men over 40 suffer from the most common form of glaucoma, according to the National Eye Institute. A simple eye exam—which looks for symptoms such as increased eye pressure and general vision deterioration— is all it takes to catch the disease early.

HEARING

Age-related hearing loss usually sets in after age 60, although it is accelerated by reckless behavior earlier in life—you know, like leaning against that bank of speakers at the Grateful Dead show in Berkeley in '86. To forestall hearing loss later in your life, keep the volume levels down when listening to music through headphones, and bring earplugs to rock concerts. The best test for gauging your hearing is also one of the oldest: the pure-tone method, which involves wearing a headset and raising your hand when you hear a sound.

HEART-RATE VARIABILITY TEST

Administered with EKG equipment, it measures the balance between the sympathetic and parasympathetic nervous systems. An overly active sympathetic nervous system indicates that you're responding poorly to stress, and may be susceptible to stress-related heart disease. A balanced reading between the two systems, on the other hand, signals that you're engaging stress in a healthy way or that those Vinyasa yoga classes are paying off.

PSA (PROSTATE-SPECIFIC ANTIGEN) TEST & DRE (DIGITAL RECTAL EXAM)

The DRE is a physical test for prostate problems in which the doctor inserts a lubed, gloved finger in your rectum to feel for bumps on the prostate gland, which should feel smooth. The PSA is a blood test that measures blood levels of the prostate-specific antigen, a protein released by prostate cells. Positive results from these tests indicate that cancer may be present, and may lead to biopsies to look for a tumor.

The PSA test was first introduced in 1987; since about 1990 when the test became a fairly routine screening for men over 40, the prostate cancer death rate has declined. But it is not clear if this drop is a direct result of the screening or due to improvements in treatment. In 2009, the *New England Journal of Medicine* published two important studies that found that screening for prostate cancer saves few lives and carries a

Self-Checks and Balances

Scheduling an annual physical doesn't mean you can ignore your body the other 364 days of the year. It's a nice idea to check in with yourself daily. Here are a couple of healthy habits to build into your life routine

FLOSS

Before you brush your teeth in the morning or at night, give your teeth a fling with the string.

Brushing alone doesn't get all the decay-causing bacteria out from between your teeth. Flossing is necessary. Plus, it's a good way to check your gum health.

Blood on your dental floss may signal gum disease, which raises the risk of heart disease and stroke. If your gums are bleeding, see your dentist.

WEIGH YOURSELF

It's a great way to keep you aware of changes in your body. Plus people who weighed themselves daily were 82 percent more likely to keep off their weight than people who didn't use a scale, according to a study at the Weight Control and Diabetes Research Center in Providence, Rhode Island.

high risk of overdiagnosis, which may lead to unnecessary treatment. (Biopsy can be painful and risky. In addition, most prostate cancers grow very slowly and may not pose a death threat.)

The American Cancer Society recommends that men of average risk over age 50, and men over age 45 with a family history of prostate cancer or who are of African heritage discuss the potential benefits and risks of screening with their doctors. "There is no debate [however] that men who have urinary symptoms, such as frequent or difficult urination, a weak stream, and so forth, ought to be getting exams including PSA tests," says Otis W. Brawley, MD, the American Cancer

SURVEY YOUR SKIN, AND FEEL FOR BUMPS

Once a week, check yourself in the mirror for moles that are asymmetrical, have changed in color, are larger than a pencil eraser, or look like the outline of Bosnia-Herzegovina (irregular borders). At least once a month, when you're in the shower, check your testicles for lumps.

POP A MULTIVITAMIN

Vitamins and minerals are best ingested through food, but there are certain nutrients that you'll need help getting even if you eat as well as Dean Ornish. In your 40s, start taking calcium and vitamin D to keep your skeleton strong.

Folic acid is so good for heart health, it's worth the extra insurance of a supplement. A good multivitamin will deliver all that and much more. It can't hurt.

SWALLOW SOME FISH OIL

"Men in their 40s and 50s can nearly reverse their risk of dying from sudden cardiac death by eating fish at least three times a week," says Joseph Hibbeln, MD, an omega-3 expert and acting chief of the section on nutritional neurosciences at the National Institutes of Health in Bethesda, Maryland. If you find it tough to get that much fish into your weekly diet,

consider taking a fish-oil supplement to reap the heart- and brain-healthy benefits of these essential fatty acids.

The American Heart Association suggests 1,000 milligrams for patients with coronary heart disease. Dr. Hibbeln believes we should consume 3,700 milligrams a day of the long-chain omega-3s EPA and DHA to balance out our high intake of omega-6s. That's the equivalent of six high-potency fish-oil capsules. You want more DHA than EPA in your supplement, about two-thirds to one-third. A prescription-only omega-3 pill called Lovaza delivers 4 grams of DHA and EPA.

Society's chief medical officer. "That's not screening. Men who have symptoms should be getting tests."

THYROID-STIMULATING HORMONE TEST (TSH)

With an overactive thyroid, there may be signs of a goiter—a swollen area in the neck. Hyperthyroidism, as it's called, can also lead to an increased heart rate, anxiety, and weight loss. Symptoms of an underactive thyroid (hypothyroidism) may include personality changes, weight gain, and a cloudy memory. Both thyroid conditions can lead to more serious, life-threatening illnesses when left untreated. The test will determine if you have a problem that a medication will remedy.

YOUR HEART:
+AN OWNER'S MANUAL

IF THERE IS ONE BODY PART to which you should devote more tender loving attention, it's the heart. The human heart is at the epicenter of your physiological and psychological universes. Not only does it keep the human body alive, it inspires the human spirit through prose and poetry, music and visual arts, and science. Edgar Allen Poe didn't write about the Telltale Kidney. When we pledge allegiance to the flag, we don't place our hand over our livers. When we get down to business, where do we start? At the heart of the matter. So, let's do just that.

Your heart is a muscle, about the size of a fist. That's important to note, because what do you do when you want to make a muscle stronger? Right, you exercise it. (File that for later.) This muscular, beating blob rests between your breastbone and spine, lovingly flanked by your lungs. It's actually three layers of muscle: the *endocardium* or smooth inner layer; the thick muscular wall, called the *myocardium*, that does the pumping; and the *epicardium* or thin membrane covering the heart, which is part of the *pericardium,* the muscle that anchors the heart to the diaphragm and major blood vessels.

Your heart is divided into four chambers, or rooms: the left atrium and right atrium at the top, and the left and right ventricles at the bottom. Like your shipping and receiving department at work, your heart is crucial to the smooth operation of the entire corporation that is your body. The atrial rooms are the receiving bays, used to collect blood from the veins as well as oxygenated blood from the lungs. With each beat, the ventricles pump blood out of the heart, either to the lungs, where it receives oxygen; or through the arteries, as it circulates to the body. That's a crucial job. Every single cell in your body requires oxygen to produce energy from food, which is why you can't survive for any extended period of time without oxygen. Your muscles need it to help you catch that bus. Your brain needs it to make heads or tails out of your stock portfolio. Your stomach needs it to digest what you just ate.

Your heart knows how and when to pump, thanks to its natural pacemaker called the sinoatrial (SA) node. The SA node is a bunch of cells in the upper-right chamber of the heart that generate electrical impulses and conduct them throughout the heart muscle, stimulating it to contract.

As you age, the impulses that trigger your heart to pump can misfire. This is what doctors call arrhythmias. The most dangerous of these is ventricular fibrillation, which causes rapid and sporadic heartbeat and inefficient blood pumping. And when oxygenated blood doesn't get to where it's needed efficiently, your brain, your lungs, your kidneys, and other organs suffer. Blood that doesn't pump out properly can pool and cause clots, triggering, you guessed it. . . .

➡ **HEART ATTACK AND HEART DISEASE** are the leading causes of death in the United States. A staggering 62 million Americans (one in every five) have some form of heart disease, and each year 960,000 men and women die of it—the equivalent of one victim every 33 seconds. (Indeed, half of the men who read this book will eventually die as a result of it—hopefully, much later in life, if you follow the advice within.) While heart disease can be ➡

Anatomy of a Heart Attack

Since the late 1990s, scientists have increasingly studied arterial inflammation to understand heart attacks. They now believe that 85 percent of heart attacks occur not when an artery clogs with fatty deposits, but when excess cholesterol inside an artery's walls incites inflammation and the growth of plaque, which then ruptures, causing a clot that blocks the blood flow to the heart. Steven E. Nissen, MD, director of the department of cardiovascular medicine of the Cleveland Clinic, explains the stages of this stealthy attack.

1

The artery wall absorbs LDL cholesterol particles, prompting cells in the wall to summon the immune system.

2

White blood cells of the immune system squeeze into the artery wall. The white blood cells emit chemical signals that cause inflammation—specifically tiny spikes on the artery called adhesion molecules, which snare more floating immune-system cells.

3

The white blood cells evolve into macrophages, which grow and ingest LDL cholesterol particles. This is the start of plaque.

4

Some of the white blood cells die and release toxins. The plaque enlarges, and the body covers it with a cap of fibrous scar tissue and muscle cells.

5

The cap ruptures, either because of a spike in blood pressure or chronic inflammation . . . no one knows for sure. The plaque—a mix of fat molecules, cholesterol, and dead white blood cells—seeps out of the wound into the artery. This attracts red blood cells, which form a clot, blocking the artery and triggering a heart attack.

triggered by many different factors, including congenital defects and infections, the leading cause is coronary artery disease, also called cardiovascular disease, also called arteriosclerosis. Call it what you will, it is worthy of your attention, and it's good to know the factors that increase your risk.

➡ **ARTERIOSCLEROSIS** is the name for a number of arterial disorders that result in the narrowing and hardening of the arteries over time. One of the main causes of arterial narrowing is **atherogenesis,** or the deposit of fats in the inner walls of the arteries. These waxy deposits are called plaque and are made up of a combination of fats, cholesterol, cell waste products, and proteins.

Like all the rest of the cells and organs in the body, the heart itself needs oxygen, which is brought to it by the coronary arteries. If the coronary arteries are blocked, then the heart doesn't get enough oxygen. The result is chest pain that you feel when you're exerting yourself, which is called **angina.** People say angina feels like a squeezing sensation, or a heavy weight settling onto their chest, although it sometimes feels like indigestion or back pain. The pain usually eases off when you stop the exertion. But it shouldn't be ignored; this is a serious early warning sign that your coronary arteries are already pretty badly compromised. Your doctor will prescribe medications to treat your angina—some to use when an attack is acute, and some to treat the underlying problem.

If your pain is severe enough or doesn't respond to medication, your cardiologist may recommend a surgical solution. During an **angioplasty,** your cardiac surgeon will expand the diameter of an artery by blowing up a very small balloon inside it. Often, a stent, which looks like a tiny metal straw, is introduced at the same time, to prevent the artery from collapsing again.

If the angioplasty doesn't work, you may need a **bypass:** Your cardiac surgeon will effectively create a detour around the blockage, using another one of your blood vessels. This is, as you might imagine, a major operation. Your heart is stopped, and a machine feeds oxygenated blood to your organs. After the operation is complete the heart is re-started. Bypass can buy angina sufferers a great deal of long-lasting relief from pain.

Plaque deposits reduce the inside diameter of the artery, causing what is, in effect, a cardiac plumbing problem. But these plaque deposits also interact with the walls of the artery, creating a lesion, so that the buildup occurs *inside* the artery walls. (See Anatomy of a Heart Attack, page 246). These lesions sometimes rupture, causing blood to clot in the area. That blood clot can cause an obstruction, leading to a heart attack or stroke. When the latter occurs, the brain is starved of oxygen, and part of it may die, leading to paralysis, language and vision loss, and other problems. The risk factors for stroke are almost identical to the ones for heart disease.

Another common heart disorder is **arrhythmia.** Some people's hearts beat with an irregular rhythm; others beat too fast, or too slow. They are all arrhythmias. You might feel your heart racing in your chest, lightheadedness, shortness of breath, or sweat more than usual. Arrhythmia becomes more and more common with age. There are many different types, and many of them are nothing more than a nuisance; but if you experience missed heartbeats or a slow or racing heart, you should get in touch with your doctor, as an irregular heartbeat can be a sign of something more serious. There's a wide range of potential causes, including damage to the heart muscle after a heart attack, abnormal hormone levels, and some medicines. If the condition is serious, your doctor will recommend medications or a pacemaker device, which uses electrical current to regulate your heartbeat.

Are You At Risk?

A number of risk factors make it more likely that you'll suffer from heart disease. As you will see, some are things completely out of your control—factors like your family history, your age, race, and sex. Others have everything to do with what you do— how well you control your health through diet, exercise, lifestyle, and medications. If you fall into some risk categories outside of your control, it will be especially important to act

HEART ATTACK WARNING SIGNS

+ Pressure, fullness, or a squeezing pain in the center of your chest that lasts for more than a few minutes

+ Pain extending beyond your chest to your shoulder, arm, back, or even to your teeth and jaw

+ Increasing episodes of chest pain

+ Prolonged pain in the upper abdomen

+ Shortness of breath

+ Sweating

+ Impending sense of doom

+ Fainting

+ Nausea and vomiting

WHAT YOU SHOULD DO IF YOU THINK YOU'RE HAVING A HEART ATTACK

➡ **Call 911.** You'll get faster treatment at most emergency rooms if you arrive by ambulance, and the paramedics can begin treating you while en route. If you don't have access to emergency services, get someone to drive you. Don't drive yourself unless it's your only option.

➡ **Chew an aspirin.** While you're waiting for the ambulance, chew and swallow a regular aspirin to speed the blood-thinning medicine to your bloodstream.

➡ **Get comfortable.** Loosening your collar and sitting in a comfortable position—often with knees bent—may allow you to breathe more easily.

---

upon the ones you can control. Let's review the risk factors.

➡ **DIABETES:** People with diabetes are two to four times more likely to suffer from cardiovascular disease. Keeping your blood sugar, cholesterol, and blood pressure at healthy levels can help you manage the risk.

➡ **FAMILY HISTORY:** If your father or mother or brother or sister— or even Uncle Danny—had heart disease, your risk rises. But a 2006 Swedish study suggests it's your mom you need to worry about more than anyone else. While your risk increases by 17 percent if your father has heart disease, it shoots up to 43 percent if your mother is afflicted. This may be due more to environment than genetics, since children typically spend more time with their mothers and are more likely to learn lifestyle habits from them. But even if you don't smoke and do exercise, it's possible that your risk could still be up as much as 82 percent if both of your parents had heart disease. Find out as much as you can about heart disease in your family—how many people had it, when they were diagnosed, and when they died. Write it down, make a copy, and give one to your doctor to leave in your file. It's important that he or she knows your family history in order to initiate preventive treatments even if you don't have any other cardiovascular disease (CVD) risk factors or symptoms.

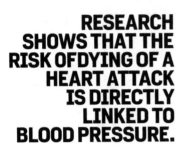

RESEARCH SHOWS THAT THE RISK OF DYING OF A HEART ATTACK IS DIRECTLY LINKED TO BLOOD PRESSURE.

➡ **HYPERLIPIDEMIA** [elevated LDL (bad) cholesterol, low HDL (good) cholesterol, high triglycerides (blood fats)]: Too much cholesterol can build up along the walls of your arteries; excess buildup blocks the flow of blood and can also invade the inside of your arteries, which can lead to instability and the possibility of a heart attack.

➡ **HYPERTENSION:** Uncontrolled high blood pressure is a direct cause of heart disease, heart attack, and stroke. In fact, research shows that the risk of dying from a heart attack is directly linked to blood pressure—the higher your blood pressure, the higher your risk, even when it's within in the normal range.

➡ **OVERWEIGHT/OBESITY:** A Body Mass Index (BMI) over 25 increases your risk for heart disease, particularly when it goes over 30. And it's not just a question of carrying too much weight. (To determine your BMI, see page 23.) *Where* you pack on the pounds seriously affects your heart disease risk (as well as your risk of stroke, diabetes, and high blood pressure, too). People with apple-shaped bodies (bodies with a lot of fat deposited around the middle) are at higher risk than those with a pear-shaped bodies (excess weight in the hips and thighs). Your doctor may measure your waist-to-hip ratio, but you can determine your risk at home. If your waist circumference (measured right above your belly button) is more than 40 inches (for men; 35 inches for women), you're at significantly increased risk for heart disease and metabolic syndrome.

➡ **RACIAL GROUPS:** African Americans, Mexican Americans, and Hawaiian Americans are at higher risk.

➡ **SEDENTARY LIFESTYLE:** Watching *Dancing with the Stars* does not constitute active living. A slothful lifestyle increases the likelihood of other risk factors—diabetes, gaining weight, high cholesterol—that put you in the path of heart disease. Exercise is strongly correlated to heart health, and, as you'll see, even a little can make a big difference.

➡ **SMOKING:** According to the American Heart Association, you increase your risk of developing coronary heart disease between two and four times, by smoking. (Just hanging out with a smoker increases your risk of heart disease, too.) And smoking multiplies other risk factors—so if your dad died of a heart attack and your cholesterol is high, smoking sends your risk profile Mount-Everest high. Smoking is also an independent risk for sudden cardiac death—a smoker is twice as likely as a nonsmoker to drop dead. If you're still smoking, quitting now is the best thing you can do to save your heart.

Keep Your Heart in Good Shape

Heart disease, high blood pressure, high cholesterol, insulin resistance, and being overweight are all interrelated with the prominent diseases that begin to show up at 40+. Fortunately, what you do to improve one symptom often improves one or more of the others. So, the benefits of a little troubleshooting rise quickly and exponentially. Here are 15 ways to do your heart good.

+ **Lower Your Blood Pressure.** Only about a third of the people with high blood pressure have it under control. That's surprising when you consider how useful this warning sign can be: Having hypertension gives you a twofold-to-fourfold increase in your risk of stroke or heart attack. Having a big belly makes your heart work harder than it has to. Here's what to do about it. One of the best things you can do to slash high blood pressure is to lose weight. In fact, bringing your weight into the normal range for your age and body type can produce a 10- to 29-point drop in blood pressure; that alone is enough of an improvement to eliminate the need to take drugs for the problem.

➡ **WATCH THE SALT.** Sodium causes your body to retain water, which increases blood volume and consequently blood pressure. Even if you don't salt your food, you are probably getting much more salt from the processed foods you eat than you need in a day. Americans average 4,000 milligrams (mg) of sodium daily, 1,600 mg more than the recommended limit. Studies show that the more sodium you eat, the shorter your life. But cutting down on salty foods can have a dramatic impact. Researchers at the University of Helsinki reviewed more than a dozen studies and found that people who reduced their sodium intake by 30 percent lived an average of 7 years longer than those whose sodium intake remained high.

Focus on eliminating the biggest salt sources in your diet. Those are processed foods like canned soups, condiments, flavored rice dishes, frozen dinners, and most fast foods. One frozen dinner can contain as much as 2,000 mg sodium, a cup of cottage cheese packs 918 mg, and a single slice of deli ham packs 240 mg. If you tend to use a salt shaker, mix up a DIY salt substitute. Australian scientists determined that diluting regular salt with potassium salt and Epsom salt (magnesium sulfate) lowers arterial blood pressure by six points. Cooking with that concoction reduces overall sodium intake and boosts blood levels of potassium, a nutrient that naturally regulates blood pressure. Pour 65 percent table salt, 25 percent Morton Salt Substitute (potassium chloride), and 10 percent Epsom salt into a small bowl, mix well, and funnel into a salt shaker. You won't taste the difference.

➡ **FIX IT WITH POTASSIUM.** The average man in his 40s gets about 3,100 mg of potassium a day, roughly 300 mg shy of the recommended amount. Making sure you regularly eat potassium-rich foods can help keep your blood pressure from climbing. Add half a can of beans, a banana, or a handful of raisins to your daily diet. Each will increase your potassium intake by about 400 mg a day, boosting you above that 3,500 mg benchmark. Beans offer a dual benefit. In the National Health and Nutrition Examination Survey, scientists found that people who consumed beans were 23 percent less likely to have large waists than those who said they never ate them. Beans are rich in belly-filling fiber as well as blood-pressure-lowering potassium. Aim for a half-cup of cooked legumes at least three times a week.

➡ **ADD STRENGTH TRAINING TO AEROBIC WORKOUTS.** You can achieve up to a 10-point drop in blood pressure from regular exercise, according to several studies. Blood vessels well trained by regular aerobic exercise expand and contract easily, which helps control blood pressure, even during times of heightened stress. And resistance exercise raises your blood pressure, which gives your body practice in bringing it back down. Researchers at the University of Michigan found that men who performed three total-body weight workouts a week for 2 months lowered their blood pressure readings by an average of eight points.

➡ **KEEP "HAPPY HOUR" SHORT.** Doctors say that once you have more than two alcoholic beverages a day, you begin to incur complications, such as an increased risk of high blood pressure. No one is quite sure why an excessive amount of alcohol, which dilates blood vessels, can sometimes raise blood pressure, but it does. If you drink, add Bloody Mary to the red wine on your healthiest-booze list. According to a study in the *American Heart Journal,* the antioxidant lycopene in tomato juice can boost your beverage's blood-pressure-lowering power. (Use the low-sodium variety for your mixer!) When participants in the study swallowed tomato-juice extract for 8 weeks, they experienced a 10-point drop in their systolic BP and a 4-point fall in their diastolic measure. Add a stalk of celery for extra protection. High in fiber, celery has been used for centuries in Asian medicine to drop blood pressure.

If you try these natural blood pressure remedies and your readings are still 20 to 30 points out of normal range, you may be genetically predisposed to hypertension and should consult your doctor about a pharmaceutical solution. Prescription drugs like diuretics ("water pills"), calcium channel blockers, inhibitors of angiotensis converting enzyme (ACE inhibitors) and alpha-adrenergic blockers are effective at bringing blood pressure into the normal range.

+ **Elevate Your HDL**. HDL acts like arterial Drano, picking up excess cholesterol from the artery walls and carting it to the liver for removal from the body. "HDL hasn't gotten the same attention as total cholesterol levels or LDL partly because there haven't been good medicines for raising it," says Daniel J. Rader, MD, an associate professor of medicine and pathology at the University of Pennsylvania School of Medicine. But HDL deserves your vigilance. Many patients with heart disease do not have elevated total cholesterol or LDL, but they do have low HDL. "It's a major coronary risk factor and a big unmet medical need," says Rader.

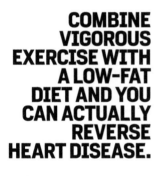

COMBINE VIGOROUS EXERCISE WITH A LOW-FAT DIET AND YOU CAN ACTUALLY REVERSE HEART DISEASE.

The National Cholesterol Education Program's updated clinical guidelines now call HDL levels "low" when they are less than 40 mg/dL. What's more, HDL levels that are 60 mg/dL and higher are now considered to be protective against heart disease.

"The higher the better," explains Roger D. Blumenthal, MD, director of the Ciccarone Preventive Cardiology Center at the Johns Hopkins University School of Medicine, in Baltimore. "It's not easy to elevate HDL [levels], but there are some effective lifestyle changes you can make; that's the cornerstone of heart disease prevention."

Following are natural techniques to try for boosting HDL. Your reward: You slash your risk of developing heart disease 2 percent for every one-point increase in HDL above 35 mg/dL, which is a benefit more dramatic than what you achieve by lowering LDL by one point.

➡ **LOSE 10 POUNDS.** Studies show that for every pound of fat you lose, your HDL rises 1 percent, so a 10-pound loss would translate into a 10-percent reduction in heart disease.

➡ **DRINK ORANGE JUICE.** A flavonoid in oranges called hesperidin may improve blood levels of HDL, says Elzbieta Kurowska, PhD, a researcher at the University of Western Ontario, in London, Ontario, Canada. In her study, 16 men were asked to drink three 8-ounce glasses of orange juice a day. After 4 weeks, blood tests revealed that their HDL had risen 21 percent (or about 10 points) from pretest levels and kept rising to a total of 27 percent after they stopped drinking the juice.

Tired of OJ? Try **cranberry.** In a study at the University of Scranton, in Pennsylvania, 19 volunteers with high cholesterol started drinking cranberry juice cocktail—8 ounces a day for the first month, then 16 ounces a day for the second month, and 24 ounces a day for the third month. A comparison of blood tests performed before and after the experiment revealed that the volunteers' HDL levels had shot up by an average of 10 percent.

➡ **BREAK A SWEAT.** In a study at Auburn University, men ages 35 to 50 who exercised 30 to 45 minutes a day for 4 consecutive days increased their HDL levels by four to six points. Other research suggests that the more intense the exercise, the better: A group of physicians training for the Boston Marathon some years ago boosted their HDL from an average of 45 to 55, according to William Castelli, MD, renowned medical director of the Framingham Cardiovascular Institute, in Massachusetts, and former director of the Framingham Heart Study.

Combine the vigorous exercise regimen with a low-fat diet, and you actually reverse heart disease, according to German researchers. In a yearlong study, men who both exercised and ate healthily saw their HDL levels climb, and 32 percent of the men with heart disease experienced a reduction in existing blockages in their coronary arteries.

➡ **GET YOUR SPOUSE TO QUIT SMOKING.** In a study at Florida State University, researchers found that exposing nonsmoking

STROKE WARNING SIGNS

+ Sudden numbness or weakness of the face, arm, or leg, especially on one side of the body

+ Sudden confusion, trouble speaking or understanding

+ Sudden trouble seeing with one or both eyes

+ Sudden, severe headache with no known cause

+ Sudden trouble walking, dizziness, loss of balance or coordination

WHAT YOU SHOULD DO IF YOU THINK YOU'RE HAVING A STROKE

➡ **Call 911.** If you or someone with you has one or more of these signs, immediately call 911.

➡ **Check the time** so you'll know when the first symptoms appeared: A clot-busting drug called tissue plasminogen activator (tPA) can reduce long-term disability for the most common type of stroke, but it has to be given within 3 hours of the onset of symptoms.

volunteers to the amount of cigarette and cigar smoke in a typical tavern depressed their HDL levels by 10 to 20 percent for 24 to 48 hours. If you live with a smoker, your HDL will be lower just from breathing. While they can't rule out the effects of the carbon monoxide in the smoke, researchers believe that nicotine is a big contributor to depressing HDL. Another study found that smokers who had used the nicotine patch to kick the habit still had low HDL levels after a month off cigarettes. But their HDL levels normalized after the patch was removed.

+ **Lower Triglycerides**. Exercise helps increase the efficiency of an enzyme called lipoprotein lipase, which attacks triglycerides and makes more HDL. Since lipoprotein-lipase levels peak about 12 hours after you exercise, it's not a bad idea to work out in the morning before, say, a big steak dinner that you know is coming in the evening. Eating a high-fat meal (or drinking a lot of booze) will flood the bloodstream with triglycerides. Prepare for that with a lipoprotein-lipase defense that can raise your HDL by 4 points.

➡ **TRY TAI CHI AND GREEN TEA.** A study in the *Journal of Alternative and Complementary Medicine* suggests that doing tai chi movements regularly can significantly raise HDL levels. Researchers asked 76 people to practice tai chi for 50-minute sessions, three times a week. After 12 weeks, the subjects' HDL levels had risen by almost 5 points. Researchers believe this benefit may be due to a change in body-fat ratio and a decrease in triglyceride levels. After a workout, drink green tea. A daily dose of the green tea extract has been shown to boost HDL by up to 4.4 percent, or more than 2 points.

✦ **Fight Inflammation.** The three triggers that stoke inflammation are LDL cholesterol, triglycerides, and an amino acid called homocysteine. When these substances are elevated in the blood, they infiltrate the artery walls and start to oxidize, or decay. Your immune system recognizes these decaying bits as a health threat and sends immune cells to consume them. These immune cells become bloated and then combine, resulting in fatty plaque filled with both cholesterol and the debris from immune cells that form inside the inflamed arteries.

Inflammation is a silent killer. You can't see it or feel it until it blossoms into heart disease. But there are biological signs that indicate its presence. One of the best-known is C-reactive protein. A simple blood test from your doctor called a CRP test (described in "A New Generation of Cardiac Tests on page 238) measures the amounts of this protein in your blood. In landmark studies reported in the *New England Journal of Medicine*, researchers at Harvard Medical School and Boston's Brigham and Women's Hospital found that people with high levels of this blood marker for inflammation are as likely as those with high cholesterol to die from a heart attack or stroke.

"The CRP test can predict risk years in the future," says Paul M. Ridker, MD, PhD, director of the Center for Cardiovascular ➡

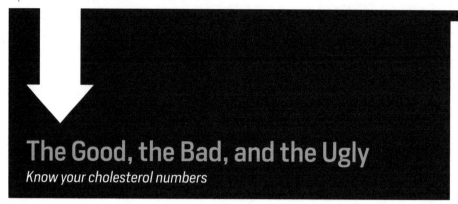

The Good, the Bad, and the Ugly
Know your cholesterol numbers

Ask your doctor to test your HDL, LDL, and total cholesterol levels, plus triglycerides (another blood fat). A high triglyceride level appears to be an especially strong predictor of heart disease in people with low HDL.

HDL (THE GOOD)	LDL (THE BAD)	TOTAL CHOLESTEROL	TRIGLYCERIDES (THE UGLY)
➡ **Optimal** 60 mg/dL or higher	➡ **Optimal** Less than 100 mg/dL	➡ **Desirable** Less than 200 mg/dL	➡ **Normal** Less than 150 mg/dL
➡ **Low** Less than 40 mg/dL	➡ **Near optimal** 100-129 mg/dL	➡ **Borderline high** 200-239 mg/dL	➡ **Borderline high** 150-199 mg/dL
	➡ **Borderline high** 130-159 mg/dL	➡ **High** 240 mg/dL or higher	➡ **High** 200-499 mg/dL
	➡ **High** 160-189 mg/dL		➡ **Very high** 500 mg/dL or higher
	➡ **Very high** 190 mg/dL or higher		

Disease Prevention at Brigham and Women's. "It opens up multiple new ways to prevent and treat cardiovascular diseases."

You can do much to intervene in the inflammatory chain reaction that creates heart disease, because so many of the triggers of inflammation are lifestyle related: carrying excess weight, eating a diet high in animal protein, smoking cigarettes, having high blood sugar, and not exercising enough. Here are six steps you can take today to douse the deadly flames.

➡ **GO FOR A WALK.** In a study at the Cooper Institute in Dallas, 722 men walked on treadmills to determine their fitness levels. It turned out that the more fit a man was, the less C-reactive protein was found in his blood. Even men who were just slightly more fit than the most sedentary guys in the study were 57 percent less likely to have elevated CRP levels. Thirty minutes of moderate exercise, 5 days a week, is a good place to start to keep your CRP low, suggest researchers at the Cooper Institute.

➡ **KEEP BLOOD SUGAR IN CHECK.** Do that naturally by avoiding refined foods like white bread and rice, fast-absorbing carbohydrates that increase the level of sugar (glucose) in the blood. "If you have high glucose in the bloodstream, it causes oxidative damage, and in response to that, there's inflammation," explains Cyril W. C. Kendall, PhD, a research scientist at the University of Toronto. To manage blood sugar, choose foods that break down into sugar slowly, such as whole wheat breads and pastas, chickpeas, most vegetables, nuts, and legumes.

➡ **HAVE GREEN TEA WITH BREAKFAST.** Studies show that your morning cup of coffee can raise CRP levels by as much as 30 percent. Substitute it with a cup of green tea (packed with phytochemicals known as polyphenols, which inhibit cancer-causing chemicals in the bloodstream) or orange juice, which is loaded with vitamin C. The latter antioxidant attacks the highly volatile oxygen molecules that are a by-product of metabolism and have been closely linked to inflammation.

➡ **ORDER THE CURRIED CHICKEN.** UCLA researchers studying the health benefits of curcumin, the yellow pigment found in the curry spice turmeric, say that it can offset the oxidative damage and inflammation that can occur deep within the brain and which is associated with Alzheimer's disease. Other studies show that the neurodegenerative disease affects only 1 percent of people over age 65 living in some Indian villages. Coincidence?

➡ **MASTER MORE EGGPLANT AND ZUCCHINI RECIPES.** The skin of the purple eggplant is rich in nasunin and chlorogenic acid, two of the most potent free-radical scavengers found in plant tissues.

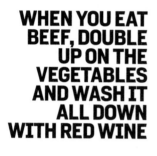

WHEN YOU EAT BEEF, DOUBLE UP ON THE VEGETABLES AND WASH IT ALL DOWN WITH RED WINE

Another benefit of eating more vegetables comes from the salicylic acid, they contain. The active ingredient in aspirin, salicylic acid is believed to moderate inflammation associated with heart disease, Alzheimer's, and cancers of the lung and colon. A study in the *Journal of Clinical Pathology* reveals that vegetarians have nearly the same levels of salicylic acid in their blood as people who pop a baby aspirin daily. This is a prime example of food as medicine. Zucchini, olives, green peppers, blackberries, cantaloupe, raisins, and cherries all contain high amounts of salicylic acid.

➡ **WASH DOWN THE STEAK WITH RED WINE.** Beef is high in stearic acid, a type of saturated fat associated with increased inflammation in your artery walls. We're not about to tell you to stop eating the occasional steak, but when you do eat it, order the petit filet, double up on the vegetables, and wash it all down with a glass of red wine. Moderate alcohol consumption is thought to reduce inflammation, and red wine is bountiful in the antioxidant chemical resveratrol. In addition, several studies show that drinking any alcohol in moderation can improve HDL levels by as much as six points.

TROUBLESHOOTING
+COMMON FITNESS-RELATED PROBLEMS

GETTING BACK INTO good physical shape sometimes comes at the price of aches, pains, and swollen joints. Here's how to troubleshoot them, and a host of other common health problems, so you can get back in the game quickly.

ACHILLES TENDONITIS

The strongest tendon in the human body—the one connecting your ankle to your calf—is only as thick as your thumb. Because it is in constant demand, it's vulnerable to injury and overload.

TREATMENT: If you feel stiffness with pain that radiates from the ankle to the calf muscle, back off your activity until you're pain-free. Ice the back of your lower leg, just above your heel, for 20 to 25 minutes every 4 to 6 hours. Strengthen and stretch the Achilles by doing lunges. Take a step forward, shift your weight onto your front foot, keeping the heel of your back foot firmly on the ground. Hold for a count of 10, return to a standing position, and then repeat the stretch with the opposite leg. Do four repetitions with each leg.

ALLERGIES

By age 40, you're probably only too familiar with your enemies—the seasonal pollens from grasses, trees, weeds, pet dander, dust mites, mold, or whatever triggers your body to release histamine. This inflammatory chemical swells the mucous membranes in your throat, nose, and eyes, making you feel as bad as your bloodshot eyes look.

TREATMENT: Avoid the enemies as best you can. Don't run outdoors in the morning when pollen counts are highest. Wear a pollen mask when you mow the lawn. And try these natural food remedies before jumping foggy-head first into drug cures:

➡ **RED ONIONS, APPLES, AND BLACK TEA** are all rich in quercetin, which inhibits production of allergy-causing histamine. But cook those onions to knock out a protein that can cause a reaction.

➡ **TURMERIC, GINGER, GARLIC, CAYENNE PEPPER, AND ROSEMARY** have anti-inflammatory properties that may reduce the swelling of the membranes that's causing your headache. **Sweet potatoes** are loaded with beta-carotene, which helps protect your airways from allergens. German researchers found that people with the highest blood levels of carotenoids—antioxidants that give fruits and vegetables their red/yellow/orange color—suffered the least from hay fever.

Walnuts are packed with alpha-linolenic acid, an omega-3 fatty acid that lessens allergy sensitivity. Walnuts also contain magnesium, which relieves constricted airways.

ASTHMA

Asthma is usually triggered by an allergy. Some irritant causes your bronchial airways to contract, you feel tightness in your chest, become short of breath, and cough and wheeze. The good news is that there's a lot you can do to get it under control.

TREATMENT: See allergy remedies above. Then try these:

➡ **AVOID RUNNING IN THE COLD.** Cold air can trigger asthma, especially when you breathe in deeply during exercise outside. If you must workout in the outdoors, cover your

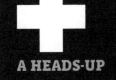

A HEADS-UP

Your Willie Is Your Heart-Health Barometer

Gentlemen: If you're having trouble maintaining an erection, it's a likely signal that your heart requires some attention. Erectile dysfunction (ED) shares several modifiable risk factors with cardiovascular disease, including atherosclerosis, hypertension, hyperlipidemia (high cholesterol, elevated triglycerides, and other blood lipid markers), diabetes, smoking, obesity, and sedentary lifestyle.

In fact, cardiologists sometimes call ED "the canary in the coal mine" because up to 75 percent of patients with chronic heart failure—an increasingly common cardiovascular disorder—report erectile dysfunction. Treat ED like the warning it is. Use it as motivation to make necessary lifestyle changes, and make sure to have your heart evaluated.

mouth and nose with a scarf or facemask. That'll help you breath in warm, humid air.

⇒ **BREATHE THROUGH YOUR NOSE.** It's estimated that one in ten people suffer from exercise-induced asthma. If you find yourself gasping for air—even while exercising in mild or warm weather outdoors—try breathing through your nose and keeping your mouth shut. Mouth-breathing draws air into the back of your throat where it dries the tissue and triggers asthma.

⇒ **BE WARY OF BEER.** Metabisulfite, found in beer, wine, shrimp, dried fruits, and some food additives, can trigger asthma. So can milk, eggs, nuts, and monosodium glutamate. Learn which foods coincide with your bouts with asthma so you can avoid them in the future.

⇒ **TAKE A DIP.** Swimming is a terrific exercise for asthmatics because the high humidity keeps your mouth from drying out. Just be aware that swimming in highly chlorinated pools without good ventilation may actually make breathing more difficult.

➡ **SHAKE THE SALT.** A recent study at Indiana University found that eating foods high in sodium can elevate the risk of exercise-induced asthma. The researchers divided 24 people with asthma into two groups—one that consumed a low-sodium diet containing about 1,500 mg per day, and another that ate a typical diet, topping out at more than 9,000 mg. (1,000 mg equals about half a teaspoon of table salt.) After exercising, those who shunned salt experienced a 20-percent improvement in lung function compared with the regular eaters. The researchers blame sodium-induced inflammation of the airways, which reduces the flow of oxygen into the bloodstream. Avoid the condition by eating fewer processed foods, which deliver up to 75 percent of our total daily salt intake.

COLDS

A cold or the flu can set your fitness routine back a week or two. Best way to beat a cold is to avoid it in the first place.

How? The vast weight of scientific evidence points to exactly one surefire strategy:

➡ **WASH YOUR HANDS.** People infected with the rhinovirus (which causes colds) transferred it to 35 percent of the surfaces they touched, where it survived for up to 18 hours, according to a recent study at the University of Virginia.

So if you've recently turned a doorknob, shaken hands, sent a fax, kissed a cheek, paid for something in cash, or otherwise interacted with the outside world, you could already have the virus at your fingertips . . . literally. You're not even safe at your desk, which, unless it's cleaned regularly, will harbor very high numbers of microorganisms, according to researchers at the University of Arizona.

➡ **EXERCISE.** While nothing comes close to preventing infection like cleanliness, another health-maintenance strategy is fitness. Moderate exercise boosts the body's production of disease-fighting white blood cells—so much so that a recent study in the journal *Medicine & Science in Sports & Exercise* found that physically active people suffered 20 percent fewer upper-respiratory infections per year than their less active counterparts.

KNEE PAIN

For a joint that's taken decades of abuse from wind sprints, jump shots, and moguls, it's surprising we're not all moving around with walkers. Knees take a lot of pressure; each time you take a step, they withstand a load many times your body weight. And if you consider their construction—akin to a bowling ball balanced on a pedestal and held in place by tight rubber bands (ligaments)—it's easy to recognize how inherently unstable they are.

But most of us take our knees for granted. They bend perfectly through thousands of steps every day, carrying us effortlessly from one destination to another. Then it happens, one wrong step, one ill-fated twist, and suddenly we're clutching crutches and wondering how such an essential joint could do us so wrong. Fortunately, most knee problems don't require surgery.

TREATMENT: Your first step after enduring a knee injury should be the RICE method—rest, ice, compression, and elevation. Wrap a bag of frozen peas or an ice pack in a towel, place it on your knee, and hold it in place relatively tightly by wrapping an elastic bandage around it. Get off your feet, and prop your leg up on pillows or an ottoman to keep the blood moving downstream, away from your knee. Do this for about 20 minutes to reduce swelling and pain.

If you don't have swelling, skip the compression and elevation parts. Many physicians recommend that their patients take an over-the-counter oral anti-inflammation medication such as Aleve or Motrin (for pain with swelling) or a painkiller like Tylenol (for pain). Your next step, however, depends on your symptoms.

➡ **IF IT HURTS TO WALK UP OR DOWN STAIRS** or to kneel or squat, you likely have **patello-femoral pain syndrome**. This is a fancy name for a multitude of problems that cause pain under or around the kneecap, including the early wearing down of cartilage (the degeneration of the lining under the kneecap) or arthritis. Patellofemoral pain syndrome is often attributed to alignment—your kneecap is higher than it should be or sits to the outside or inside of your thigh, where your muscles aren't as strong. Pain can also be from either flatfeet or ill-fitting shoes.

TREATMENT: Ice the sore spot for 20 minutes, every couple of hours, and take anti-inflammatories. Limit or stop the aggravating activity, whether it's running, playing tennis, or using the stair-climber. Also stop doing squats or lunges until the pain subsides.

➡ **IF YOU FEEL PAIN JUST BELOW THE KNEECAP,** it may be **patellar tendonitis.** It generally hurts during or after playing a sport like basketball that involves jumping, which is why this problem is also called jumper's knee. It's an overuse injury to the tendon that connects your patella, or kneecap, to your tibial tubercle, the bump on your lower-leg bone. Anytime you lift your leg (walking, jumping, raising it in the air), all of the weight of your leg goes to that point. The entire lower leg is held up by that one tendon.

TREATMENT: Rest your knee—the tendon needs time to heal. Treat it with ice and anti-inflammatories. Wearing a knee brace might also help because it takes tension off the tendon. While the injury is healing, switch to exercises that won't irritate the tendon, such as swimming or very-light-resistance cycling.

➡ **YOU HEAR A POP, THEN FEEL INTENSE PAIN.** Your knee may also buckle and give way. Chances are, you won't be able to continue whatever it was that you were doing. The likely diagnosis is a **sprained or torn ligament.** There are four ligaments in the knee—two run alongside the knee joint, while the other two crisscross inside the joint, holding it in place. The two most commonly injured are the medial collateral ligament (MCL) and the anterior cruciate ligament (ACL).

TREATMENT: Assuming you haven't injured your ACL, you'll probably do fine with a little rehab, which usually involves icing the knee and doing exercises to regain strength and stability.

If you've torn your ACL, however, more aggressive

treatment might be in order. Once it's torn, the ACL doesn't tighten and heal the way the other ligaments do. There will be a risk of knee instability, especially with high-demand sports that really challenge that ligament, such as basketball, volleyball, and soccer. If you want to continue playing high-impact sports, you'll likely benefit from arthroscopic ligament reconstruction. Afterward, it will take about 6 to 9 months to get back to aggressive activities.

➡ **IF YOU FEEL A TWINGE OR TEARING SENSATION IN THE KNEE** you may have a **torn meniscus,** the cartilage or cushioning tissue that separates the thigh bone (femur) from the larger lower-leg bone (tibia). Swelling typically follows, especially in the back of your knee. Often, a torn meniscus accompanies an ACL tear.

TREATMENT: If you don't have a locked knee from a piece of cartilage caught in the joint or an associated injury like an ACL tear, you may do very well with physical therapy alone. Some studies have shown that if you remove even a portion of the cartilage, arthritic changes occur within a few years. Avoiding surgery may be advisable. However, if you have a locked knee, typically caused by a tear known as a bucket-handle tear, then you may need arthroscopic surgery to trim the cartilage.

LOW-BACK PAIN

This is usually triggered by muscle strain. When muscles are stretched, microscopic tears occur in those fibers, which release chemicals that activate nerve endings throughout the area.

TREATMENT: Take ibuprofen, and apply heat to the area for 10 to 15 minutes a few times a day. But don't shut down things completely. Dial down your activity a bit, but don't hop into bed and avoid everything; that'll lead to stiffness and decreased flexibility, both of which will only increase the pain. Still hurts? Stretch your hamstrings once your body is already warmed up, not before. When the hamstrings are tight, they can pull on the small postural muscles of the low back, causing pain.

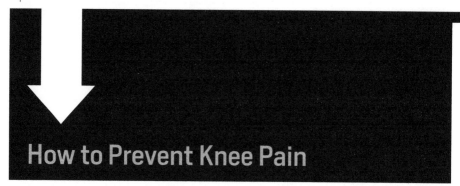

How to Prevent Knee Pain

Most knee injuries occur not because of a defect in the joint, but because of an imbalance in the muscles surrounding it—weak quads, hamstrings, or calves, for example. By increasing your quad strength and working on balance and flexibility, you can cut your risk of knee injury dramatically. Here are some ways to protect this vulnerable joint.

QUAD PUMP

When it comes to our knee joint, we're like the Tin Man from the *Wizard of Oz*—badly in need of lubrication. A lot of the dull pain we feel in our knees stems from the fact that we sit around in office chairs all day, and the joint isn't being effectively lubricated. This 10-second exercise, which could be done in your office, causes your cartilage to secrete fluid that bathes the knee joint in nutrients, keeping it healthy.

Sit in a chair and extend your legs straight out so that your heels are resting on the floor. Then tighten your quadriceps, the thigh muscles just above your knees. Hold the contraction for 2 seconds, then release. Repeat five times. Then do another set. Do quad pumps three times a day.

PLANTAR FASCIITIS

The plantar fascia is a tough thick band of fibrous tissue from the heel to the ball of the foot that helps hold up the arch. If it feels as if you've stepped on an acorn when you take your first few steps after waking up, you probably have an inflammation of this tissue, called plantar fasciitis.

TREATMENT: Ease up on the cardio until the stabbing pain's edge dulls. Also, avoid running on inclined treadmills or steep hills, which can strain the plantar fascia. Take ibuprofen, and ice your heel for 15 to 20 minutes.

Loosening up the area might also help. People with

LEG PRESS

Using a leg-press machine will help strengthen your quadriceps. The exercise places the same amount of stress on the knee that running does but in a more controlled manner. Work your legs together or separately—it doesn't matter. But aim for two sets of 10 to 12 repetitions, increasing the weight gradually as you grow stronger.

SINGLE-LEG STANCE

Stand on one leg for 30 seconds to a minute, increasing the time as you get better at holding the pose without falling. This will strengthen the muscles and ligaments around your knee as they work to stabilize the joint. You can also do these while rotating slowly to your left and right. Do two repetitions on each leg, two or three times a day.

HEEL RAISE

Stand with both heels hanging off the back of a stair or curb. Rise on your toes and hold for 5 seconds; return to starting position. This will strengthen and stretch your calf muscles. Do two repetitions, two or three times a day.

CALF STRETCH

Place one foot in front of the other and bend your knees. You should feel the stretch in the back of your lower legs. Do three repetitions, holding the stretch for 20 to 30 seconds. (Walk or jog for 5 to 10 minutes before stretching to warm up.) For another version of this stretch, see page 141.

HAMSTRING STRETCH

Place one foot on a waist-high stationary object like a chair, and slowly lean forward, reaching down the shin of the extended leg until you feel a stretch in the hamstring. Keep your back straight to avoid injury. Do three repetitions for each leg, holding the stretch for 20 to 30 seconds. For another version of this stretch, see page 121.

this problem often have tight calf muscles and Achilles tendons. Try rolling each foot over a tennis ball for 10 to 15 minutes, several times a day. You can also stand and roll your foot on a frozen golf ball or frozen water bottle to loosen the tissue.

There are many other problems that can threaten to keep you off the field, but most can be fixed with rest and ibuprofen. In the next chapter, we'll troubleshoot a different set of challenges, those that can make you look older than your body feels. Get ready to give your hair, teeth, and skin an anti-aging makeover.

chapter 9

GREAT SKIN, TEETH & HAIR AT 40+

Natural Ways For Guys to Turn Back the Clock

ONGRATULATIONS! If you've been following the advice in this book, you are already looking fitter, healthier, and younger than when you turned to page one. You know you feel better and younger, and the proof of it can no doubt be found in your bathroom mirror. But perhaps it's better to ask the opinion of an honest, unbiased observer—like your wife or partner. If you've been married for a while, odds are she will give you a candid answer, painful as it might be. If you're not married, ask a family member, like your wise-guy brother. Tell him you can handle the truth.

How can you be so sure you'll get a positive response? Well, because the most effective ways to look youthful and fight the "symptoms" that are typically associated with aging are the methods outlined in this book. When your body is fit and trim, when you're exercising, eating right, and sleeping well, you'll appear more energetic and youthful even before you try out a ➡

teeth-whitening preparation or dab some Just for Men onto those graying temples. In fact, as a reminder, here are the top seven ways to look 5 years younger in 6 weeks or less.

+ **Move!** Take brisk walks, runs, bike rides, or swims.

+ **Lose!** Take off the weight, and keep your waist trim.

+ **Eat!** Four to six small meals daily, with a variety of colorful fruits and vegetables.

+ **Workout!** Do strength-training exercises two to three times a week.

+ **Sleep!** Get 7 to 8 hours of deep, rejuvenating sleep every night.

+ **De-stress!** Manage your stress level with the tips in Chapter 6.

+ **Smile!** Keep an upward-looking, positive attitude.

Do these things first, and you will look and feel better than you have in 15 years. And people will notice.

Now, that's not to say you can't do even better. You can turn back the clock 10 years by paying a bit more attention to the three body parts that shape the first impression you deliver to the world: your teeth, skin, and hair. This chapter will provide easy, practical, mostly natural ways to make your teeth whiter, your skin smoother, and your hair thicker and more youthful.

+YOUR SKIN

NATURAL WAYS TO SMOOTH WRINKLES AND KEEP SKIN SUPPLE

LET'S START WITH SKIN, your billboard to the outside world. Skin is the largest organ of the body, measuring about 22 square feet of surface and weighing roughly 6 to 8 pounds. Your skin is composed of two layers: the epidermis, or outer layer, which is as thin as the plastic wrap on your roast beef sandwich, and the thicker dermis layer, which could be up to a half-inch thick on your back. The epidermis is your body's first line of defense. It's your cellular body armor, designed to withstand the assaults of the outside world, from sticker bushes to skin's public enemy number one—the sun.

The epidermis is made up of four layers: the stratum corneum, the outermost, which you can see and feel; the granular layer; the squamous cell layer; and the basal cell layer, where skin cells are produced. About every 30 days, your body produces a brand new epidermis, essentially allowing you the opportunity to put on a new face every month. Those skin cells manufactured in the basal layer work their way up to the top of the stratum corneum and eventually slough off, to the tune of 9 pounds of dead skin per year.

Below the epidermis, the deeper dermis layer is a combination of blood vessels, nerves, hair follicles, sebaceous (oil) glands, and two important proteins, collagen and elastin, which provide firmness and elasticity to the skin. Below all that is a layer of subcutaneous fat that softens the skin's texture. The dermis is important to the 40+ face because that's where wrinkles originate. As you get older, your skin gets thinner and drier and loses its elasticity. All that happens because collagen and elastin fibers start to break down, disrupting the skin's support structures and causing wrinkles and sags. And 80 percent of that breakdown— the changes associated with aging—is attributable to sun exposure. That's why protecting your skin from the dermis-damaging ultraviolet rays of the sun is the single most important skin care practice you can adopt. We'll start there, then suggest other easy ways to help your skin look younger.

+ **Wear sunscreen every day.** Even if you are staying indoors. As much as half of your exposure to UVA rays that cause sunspots and fine lines occurs while you're inside, according to a new study in the *Journal of Drugs in Dermatology*. The main source is light coming through windows (most glass only stops UVB rays). Get in the habit of applying a broad-spectrum sunscreen with a Sun Protection Factor (SPF) of at least 15, the higher the better. If you're going outside, reapply your sunscreen every hour to hour-and-a-half because rubbing, sweating, and swimming tend to wear off the protection. Don't forget to cover the sides of your face, the tops of your ears, and the edge where your forehead meets your hairline. Sun damage not only triggers wrinkles, but also, of course, can cause skin cancer. Each year there are more than 1 million cases of non-melanoma and 50,000 cases of melanoma skin cancer diagnosed, and roughly 10,000 deaths attributed to both. You have a nearly 50 percent chance of developing non-melanoma skin cancer at age 65 or older unless you take care of your skin now.

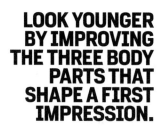

LOOK YOUNGER BY IMPROVING THE THREE BODY PARTS THAT SHAPE A FIRST IMPRESSION.

+ **Eat more cantaloupes.** National Cancer Institute researchers determined that people who consume the most carotenoids—pigments that occur naturally in plants—were as much as six times less likely to develop skin cancer as those with the lowest intakes. Beta-carotene, the antioxidant in carrots, sweet potatoes, and cantaloupes, offers internal sun protection against skin damage. That's because the vitamin plants itself directly into your skin, where its orange and yellow pigments help deflect sunlight. Eating two sweet potatoes a week will give you the same amount of beta-carotene as the men in the NCI study who demonstrated the lowest skin-cancer risk.

What About Botox?

Injectible youth comes with risks

Botox injections are a cosmetic procedure that smoothes out wrinkles by blocking the neurotransmitter acetylcholine that tells the facial muscle to contract or tense up. As the muscle relaxes, the wrinkles soften. Although the procedure was first adopted by women, hundreds of thousands of men in their 40s and older now go Bo. The problem with Botox is that it's not a once-and-done affair. You have to keep going back to the dermatologist if you want to keep the wrinkles at bay. And beware of quick fixes. New studies show that Botox's paralyzing effect has a downside: it can cause facial muscles to atrophy, resulting in skin depressions. We recommend beating wrinkles the natural way: sunscreen, sleep, and moisturizers.

+ **Keep your skin moist.** When the skin's internal scaffolding—your network of elastin and collagen fibers—starts to loosen and sag, the oil-secreting glands of the face can atrophy and rob your face of its natural lubrication. The result: premature wrinkling. But moisturizing every day can delay that for years. Apply a moisturizer in the morning as soon as you leave the shower (and before you towel yourself dry) to trap the water against your skin. Reapply at least twice more during the day and especially after a workout. And drink at least a quart of water a day to keep your skin well hydrated. Get in the habit of downing a glass of water as soon as you wake up and then before every meal and snack.

+ **Reduce your carb consumption.** A British study found that taking in 50 grams more carbohydrates (the amount in a medium order of french fries) or just 17 grams of fat per day can boost your odds of developing wrinkles by up to 36 percent—independent of both age and sun exposure.

+ **Order the salmon, papayas, and dark chocolate.** Eating foods rich in antioxidant vitamins and other healthy nutrients keeps skin supple and healthy. A study in the *American Journal of Clinical Nutrition* recently showed that people with diets rich in vitamin C decreased their odds of having fine lines and dryness by up to 11 percent. Terrific sources of vitamin C are papayas, oranges, strawberries, broccoli, and red, green, and yellow peppers.

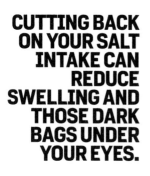

CUTTING BACK ON YOUR SALT INTAKE CAN REDUCE SWELLING AND THOSE DARK BAGS UNDER YOUR EYES.

Similarly, Korean researchers determined that omega-3 fatty acids from oily fish protected collagen from exposure to UV rays. Good food sources include salmon and sardines, as well as flaxseeds and walnuts. Selenium from food has also been shown to reduce sun damage and improve skin elasticity. Crab, wheat germ, and Brazil nuts are excellent sources of selenium.

Even dessert can improve the appearance of your skin, according to German scientists. When the researchers asked subjects to drink a cocoa beverage high in compounds called flavonols every day for 12 weeks, their skin exhibited 25 percent less damage from UV rays. The researchers believe that the antioxidants may absorb UV light and prevent inflammation as well as boost blood flow through the skin, improving texture. For the richest chocolate source of antioxidants, choose dark chocolate made with 70 percent cacao.

+ **Check your bags.** Nowhere is your skin thinner than around your eye sockets. As the years pass, skin can thin even more, allowing blood vessels beneath to show through. Then bags and dark circles start to form as the fat under the skin absorbs water. Cutting back on your salt intake can improve the situation. Too much salt in your diet can cause your body to flood with water, fattening those pouches under your eyes, so cut it out. Another effective strategy is placing chilled spoons or cotton balls dipped in a 50/50 mix of cold water and milk over your eyes in the morning for 5 minutes to reduce swelling. Or reach for an over-the-counter fix. Apply a dollop of your wife's eye cream under your eyes each night before you hit the sack. Use a serum containing topical anti-inflammatories and caffeine, which will tighten the skin into a dense layer to hide the circles.

+ **See spots run.** The brown marks on the skin that we call age spots are piles of sun-damaged dermis that have clumped together creating a blotch. Regular use of sunscreen will prevent this from happening; but if you already have them, try applying a skin cream that contains the ingredient kojic acid, or a skin-bleaching agent containing hydroquinone. If you have too many spots to take care of yourself, see a dermatologist for a laser treatment.

+ **Beat crow's feet.** An alpha hydroxy acid (AHA) such as glycolic acid is effective at stripping away the dead skin cells on your face that can make smile lines and crow's feet wrinkles more noticeable. Used once a week with an exfoliating soap, an AHA can help you flatten out the topography of wrinkled areas by accelerating cellular turnover and leaving smoother layers behind. But because it sloughs off protective skin layers, be sure to use a sunscreen as well.

+ **Sleep deep.** Sleep is one of the most important restoratives for your skin. Try to get 8 hours a night. While you're asleep, your body produces collagen and elastin, the proteins that help your skin stay smooth.

+ **Wear sunglasses.** The bigger the better—aviators or other wide-frame sunglasses with UV protection both shield the skin around your eyes from the sun and curb the squinting that creases your skin.

+YOUR TEETH

A BRIGHT SMILE CAN TAKE YEARS OFF YOUR APPEARANCE

Teeth naturally yellow as you get older—making you look older, even years older than you really are. No wonder the teeth whitening industry continues to boom to the tune of more than $500 million a year. In these tough economic times, a little cosmetic dentistry to brighten your smile or repair a chipped tooth or crooked smile could mean the difference between snagging a job or losing one. In fact, a 2008 Columbia University study found that people with healthier-looking teeth earn more than those with dull, dingy smiles. Here are some natural ways to improve the health of your teeth and gums and make them look years younger, followed by a smart approach to whitening.

+ Keep fighting cavities. Even tooth-colored composite fillings can make you look older if you have a mouth full of them. Keep your teeth looking healthy by flossing daily and brushing after every meal. Drinking cranberry juice can help prevent cavities, too. In a study at the University of Rochester, researchers exposed tooth enamel to cranberry juice and found that the acids in the juice inhibited the growth of decay-causing bacteria by 85 percent.

Having two glasses a day of a drink containing at least 25 percent cranberry-juice concentrate should keep a bacterial bloom from attacking your teeth. But be sure to drink it with meals to avoid exposing your teeth to the acid alone, which may cause the enamel to erode over time. In addition, avoid brushing your teeth immediately after drinking cranberry juice or orange juice or eating any acidic foods (oranges, grapefruit, bananas, some cereals) because brushing could remove some of the temporarily softened tooth enamel. Wait 20 minutes before you brush, experts advise.

+ **Sail the high Cs.** Making sure to eat foods rich in vitamin C and calcium will help you to keep your teeth and gums healthy looking. One study of more than 12,000 adults at the State University of New York at Buffalo found that people who got less than an orange's worth of vitamin C a day (60 mg) were 25 percent more likely to have gum disease than those who took in 180 mg or more of C.

And getting 1,000 to 1,200 mg of calcium is crucial, too. After all, 99 percent of the calcium in your body resides in your bones and teeth. The dietary calcium you get from cheese, milk, and yogurt strengthens an important bone that supports a healthy smile—the alveolar bone in the jaw, which helps hold your teeth in place.

+ **Chew celery.** Some tooth-surface stains can be eliminated simply by eating foods like apples, celery, and carrots, which contain high amounts of cellulose, a natural abrasive. Other vegetables—spinach, broccoli, and lettuce, in particular— contain mineral compounds that form a protective film over teeth so pigments from foods and drinks can't stain.

+ **Brush with baking soda.** The abrasive particles polish the surface while a chemical reaction between the baking soda and water bleaches out stains. Try it just once a week; using it more often may damage enamel. Dip a wet toothbrush in the powder before brushing, or try toothpaste that contains baking soda, such as Arm & Hammer Complete Care Toothpaste.

+ **Drink tea.** Sure, tea can stain teeth, but it has so many health benefits, even dental ones, that it's worth the offset. Black and green teas contain antioxidant plant compounds called polyphenols that prevent plaque from adhering to teeth and reduce your chances of developing cavities and gum disease. Tea also inhibits bacteria growth, which reduces bad breath.

+ **Avoid yellow shirts.** Warm-colored shirt-and-tie combos (yellows, oranges, browns, and warm shades of red) can visually

EXPERT ADVICE

Q. Should I floss before I brush my teeth, or after?

Always floss first. This will not only lessen the chance that you'll skip this vital ritual altogether, but it will also help ensure that whatever flotsam is stirred up by flossing doesn't stay in your mouth. With this sequence, you can disrupt plaque and dislodge food particles from between your teeth, which you'll then be able to sweep out more thoroughly with brushing. As for which floss to use, go with whatever type you find easiest to slip between your teeth. A dental tape may work better for tighter teeth. A study published in the *Journal of Periodontology* compared different kinds of flosses, including unwaxed, woven, and shred-resistant, and found almost no difference in their ease of use or overall effectiveness.

— **DAVID KIM, DDS, DMSC,** *an assistant professor at the Harvard School of Dental Medicine*

emphasize the yellow in your teeth. Wearing blue-based, dark, or cool-colored clothes will make the white of your teeth stand out.

+ **Pick your teeth-whitening strategy.** There are dozens of teeth-whitening options to choose from, but your biggest decision comes down to two options—doing it at home yourself or having your dentist do it. The difference is in speed, strength, and cost of the bleaching procedure. All bleaching methods use peroxide to dissolve surface stains. Since your teeth are extremely porous, they readily absorb stain-causing pigments from the foods (blueberry pie) you eat and drink (coffee, red wine, and colas). Anything that can destroy a crisp white shirt can stain your teeth.

The peroxide in teeth-whitening preparations seeps into the microscopic crevices in your teeth and lightens the stains. How fast it works depends upon the method. The whitening agents that dentists use can be three times more powerful than home versions, so you'll get quicker, more dramatic results. Typically, a protective gel or rubber barrier is placed over your gums to avoid sensitivity to the harsh peroxide. Then the teeth are coated with the bleaching agent and a light is aimed at them to foster the chemical reaction that whitens the teeth. It takes about an hour and can cost up to $800. There is a less expensive method. For $200 to $400, your dentist can fit you with a dental tray and send you home with a kit of peroxide gel tubes. You fill the tray with the gel and place it on your teeth for about half an hour a day. You'll typically see results in a week or so.

Store-bought bleaching kits work well, too. And they are much less expensive, from $15 to $50. But you should consult your dentist before trying them, because some types of dental work, such as crowns and veneers, won't take peroxide-based lighteners. And if your teeth were stained by taking an antibiotic like tetracycline in your youth, at-home brighteners won't be effective. Your dentist will be able to advise you about the best method for your teeth. When using an over-the-counter teeth whitener, coverage is key. Peroxide-infused strips and fixed trays may not adequately cover your teeth, missing the crevices in between and causing uneven bleaching. The best at-home whitening kits come with custom-moldable trays, which ensure even distribution of the bleaching chemicals.

+YOUR HAIR

ERASE AGE WITH HEALTHIER-LOOKING LOCKS

By age 50, about half of us are at least 50 percent gray. The good news is that your stressful job/family/marriage/golf game probably has little to do with it. European researchers recently discovered that graying hair is more likely due to a natural buildup of hydrogen peroxide in your hair cells. The researchers found that this buildup over time blocks synthesis of a natural hair pigment. So, essentially, the hair bleaches itself from the inside out. Stress still may have something to do with it, but clearly genetic factors play a role in who will become gray and when.

We'll talk about the color fix for this in just a bit, but graying hair isn't the only reality of aging that contributes to adding years to your appearance. Dry hair, thinning hair, balding, even dandruff can also make you look older than you really are. But just as you can get your muscles to respond to exercise, there is much you can do to improve the look of what you've got up top, even for you guys who may have very little of it. Consider the following a circuit workout for your locks.

+ **Deal with dandruff.** White flakes on your suit jacket make you look careless and unkempt. And it's avoidable, since dandruff in its many variations is highly treatable with over-the-counter or prescription shampoos and creams. But let's start by trying some easy home remedies. Before bedtime, dampen your scalp with a little warm water to open the pores and then rub a capful of baby oil into your scalp. The oil will seep into your scalp and soften up the dandruff scales, loosening them enough that they will fall off when you shower the next morning.

Another home treatment that some people find effective is apple cider vinegar. Apply it from a spray bottle or simply pour a little over your head in the shower. The vinegar acts as a fungicide to fight the cause of the cell buildup as well as a rinsing agent. Honey is another natural antifungal. In one study, dandruff sufferers who prewashed their scalps daily with honey diluted with warm water had no more flakes or itching after 5 weeks.

There also are dozens of anti-dandruff shampoos on the market that are effective against mild dandruff. The gold standard is a tar shampoo containing salicylic acid, the active ingredient in aspirin. The mild acid restores normal acidity to the scalp, breaking down the oils that lead to clumping and flaking. Since dandruff varies from person to person, you may have to try a number of different shampoos to find the one that works best for you. Neutrogena T/Gel contains coal tar; Selsun Blue uses the active ingredient selenium sulfide; and Head & Shoulders and Redken For Men Retaliate anti-dandruff shampoo contain zinc pyrithione and won't leave your scalp smelling like a medicine cabinet. If you have a severe case of dandruff due to seborrheic dermatitis, try a shampoo containing 2 percent ketoconazole, such as Nizoral. Here's a hint from experienced guys: Some dandruff sufferers find that switching between different types of anti-dandruff shampoos every few weeks works best. For persistent dandruff that doesn't improve, see a dermatologist for a prescription-strength shampoo or cream.

+ Get into condition. Mature hair is often a lot drier and coarser than the kind you find on a 5-year-old. But you can soften and add shine to your rugged mop with a simple moisturizing shampoo. Women already know this, so somewhere in the house you'll be able to find some of this shampoo or a conditioner. Give it a try, and then find your own. For especially dry and coarse hair, try a moisturizing shampoo or conditioner containing wheat-germ oil, shea butter, or nut oils. If you have the opposite problem, oily hair, try a conditioner containing oil-absorbing tea-tree oil. Men with fine or thin hair should avoid conditioners, which may weigh down hair follicles. Try a hair-thickening shampoo containing the body-building ingredient panthenol to make hair strands thicker.

+ **Choose the right cut.** When it comes to length, there is no argument. Shorter equals younger, especially if your hair is thinning. The light, bouncy effect of a good short haircut will make your hair look fuller. One of the best techniques for disguising thinning hair is to let the hair on top of the head grow out a bit while reducing bulk at the back and sides. Find a good barber. A hairstylist with experience will work with a person's natural features and the part, texture, and wave of the hair to create an attractive and easy-to-maintain style. A good sign is a hairstylist who favors scissors over electric clippers. Scissors create a texturized cut that varies the length of the hair strands. When you add a grooming product to texturized hair, the staggered ends will form scaffolding that will support the weight of the hair so it won't fall flat.

+ **Lose the beard.** Facial hair, especially beards, adds years to a man's appearance. If you've had facial hair for a long time, try shaving it off during a 2-week vacation, and see if you don't look younger. Ask your wife or girlfriend for confirmation. You can always grow it back by the time you return to work.

+ **Color your gray.** If you're considering coloring your hair, first see a colorist at your barbershop or hairstylist. The best salons have people who specialize in hair color, and it is worth spending more for a good one. Amateur or at-home hair dye will often leave you with a flat, unnatural, single-color look with no highlights, which makes you look, frankly, kinda desperate. And when choosing a color, select one that's a shade or two lighter than your natural hair color. This way you'll achieve a more natural blend that won't look so stark and dramatic.

+ **Don't forget the brows.** Eyebrows should match your hair color. If you color your hair, have a pro do your eyebrows to avoid getting the chemicals in your eyes. And whenever you have your hair trimmed, have the barber trim your eyebrows. Bushy, unruly eyebrows will make you look like Andy Rooney— or a crazy old scientist.

+ **Handle hair loss.** Today men have a number of FDA-approved non-surgical treatments for androgenetic alopecia, more commonly known as male-pattern baldness. Some work better than others, and you may have to try several to determine the best for you.

➡ MINOXIDIL: Marketed as Rogaine by McNeil-PPC, minoxidil started out as a blood-pressure pill that seemed to grow hair. It's now the only topical preparation approved by the FDA for male-pattern hair loss. Doctors believe that it works by dilating blood vessels in the scalp, triggering hair to grow longer and thicker. Minoxidil is applied twice a day, and you have to use it for life. There's a generic version that's about 30 percent less expensive than McNeil's Rogaine. Some dermatologists believe adding Retin-A (which contains the acid form of vitamin A, tretinoin) enhances treatment by making the top layers of skin in the scalp more permeable, which aids in the absorption of minoxidil.

➡ FINASTERIDE: This drug, marketed as Propecia and other brands, works by inhibiting the formation of dihydrotestosterone (DHT), a hormone that shrinks hair follicles. It is also able to trigger new hair growth in some patients, especially those in the earliest stages of hair loss. The pill must be taken daily for life. Finasteride was initially developed as a prescription drug to treat englarged prostates, a common disorder called benign prostatic hyperplasia, or BPH. Marketed as Proscar, the BPH drug contains 5 mg finasteride. So, to save money over the more expensive Propecia (a 1-mg pill), you can ask your doctor to prescribe Proscar, then use a pill splitter to divide the drug into four pieces and take one-quarter of the pill a day.

➡ LASERS: A handheld device called the HairMax Lasercomb administers low-level laser therapy to the scalp, supposedly to energize the mitochondria or "power plants" in cells. It is believed that this may trigger dormant hair follicles to grow again in 3 to 4 months of use during 10-minute sessions, three times a week. The $500 device has been approved by the FDA. However, it should be noted that the FDA approval process is less stringent with devices than with drugs.

chapter 10

THE 40+ MEDICINE CABINET

Even a Fit Body Can Benefit From a Little Drugstore Help Now and Then

SEVERAL YEARS BACK the British Museum in London showcased a contemporary art installation called *Cradle to Grave*, by a doctor and two artists who call themselves Pharmacopoeia. The piece, which explores the modern approach to healthcare, incorporates a lifetime's supply of prescription drugs sewn into two, 43-foot-long textiles, each length containing more than 14,000 pills, tablets, and capsules, the estimated average number prescribed to every Brit during his or her lifetime. And that doesn't include over-the-counter remedies or nutritional supplements, which would amount to another 40,000 doses.

If that sculpture were made in the United States, New York City's Museum of Modern Art would need to expand half a block on to Sixth Avenue: Americans are by far the most medicated society in the world. According to IMS Health, which tracks the pharmaceutical industry, the United States accounts for　➡

$291 billion of the estimated $450 billion total worldwide annual sales for prescription drugs. The average American fills 12.6 prescriptions a year, up from 8.9 a little over 10 years ago. From 1997 to 2007, the number of total prescriptions filled in the United States increased 66 percent, to 3.5 billion annually. And those figures don't take into account drugs dispensed by hospitals, clinics, and doctors' offices. Add to that the tens of billions of doses of over-the-counter remedies we take per year. For perspective, Americans consume nearly 20 million aspirin tablets every single day.

AMERICANS CONSUME NEARLY 20 MILLION ASPIRIN TABLETS EVERY SINGLE DAY.

More and more public health experts, researchers, and even doctors are coming to the conclusion that America is over-dosing on medicine, buying and taking too much, too carelessly, in the pursuit of fast relief. We're not advocating that you toss out your ACE inhibitors and Excedrin—some drugs are lifesavers, and OTC medications can make bad colds and everyday aches much more bearable. But if you're like most Americans, you can probably do just as well without popping a pill for every niggling health glitch. As often as you can, let your body's immune system do its job, and selectively take only the medicines that will greatly benefit you. To help you self-regulate your self-medicating, here's a guide to getting the right OTC stuff for what ails you.

Over-the-Counter Medications

We've all been there. Standing in the fluorescent light of the cold-remedy aisle of a 24-hour pharmacy at 2 a.m., sinuses pounding, throat on fire, shivering and hacking while we gaze at a dizzying array of syrups, elixirs, capsules, and tabs. In a survey by the National Council on Patient Information and Education, 66 percent of adults said that picking the right non-prescription drug was a daunting task. Not surprising when you consider that there are more than 100,000 OTC meds on the market. So, how do you choose from 60 or more cold and flu drugs, pain relievers, and allergy medicines in the cold-remedy aisle when you need relief fast? Better to plan ahead and stock your medicine cabinet with these tried-and-true remedies for life's most common minor health problems.

ACHES AND PAINS
➡ Fight back with **ibuprofen.**

It's the best OTC medication for pain associated with swelling and inflammation. According to a recent study published in the *Journal of Rheumatology*, osteoarthritis sufferers preferred ibuprofen over acetaminophen two to one.

Start with 200 mg four times a day, and if that doesn't help, you can go up to 400 mg. Look for Advil, Motrin, or generic ibuprofen. Studies show that liquid ibuprofen or capsules containing dissolved ibuprofen are absorbed into the bloodstream 50 percent quicker than standard tablets.

ALLERGIES
➡ Fight back with **Claritin.**

The reason you're sneezing, your nose is running, your eyes are watering, and you look and feel awful is that allergens in the air have invaded your nasal passages and triggered your immune system to release histamine, an inflammatory compound. The antihistamine loratadine found in Claritin blocks histamine to prevent all that from making you feel miserable.

Diphenhydramine, the antihistamine in Benadryl and other antihistamine preparations, can cause drowsiness. Claritin doesn't, at least not as much. A 2005 study by researchers at the Washington Neuropsychology Research Group in Washington, D.C., found that seasonal allergy sufferers who took Claritin were as alert and focused as those participants who didn't have allergies.

Keep in mind that a common sidekick of allergies is headache. This medicine won't help that symptom. If you have a headache, take a pain reliever like aspirin.

ATHLETE'S FOOT
➡ Fight back with **terbinafine, tolnaftate, and miconazole nitrate.**

Fungal infections on the skin start in warm, moist places, which is to say usually between your toes, or between your legs, where it's known as jock itch. The fungus is the same in both places, and the way to get rid of it is with a cream-based antifungal like LamisilAT (terbinafine hydrochloride), Tinactin (tolnaftate), or Micatin (miconazole nitrate). It'll usually clear up within a week or two.

Since the fungus can build up immunity to any one kind of medication, it's a good idea to have two or more different brands on hand, and alternate them daily. (Yes, you are now in a battle of wits with fungus.)

COLD SORES
➡ Fight back with **Abreva.**

Feel that tingling on your upper lip? It could be the start of a cold sore that may erupt into a lesion the size of a paperweight in a few days. A cold sore is typically a recurrence of herpes simplex virus type 1, which is something you picked up somewhere along the line and has been lying dormant in the nerve cells in your skin.

Cold sores are highly contagious and tend to recur under some form of physical or mental stress. Recurrence is usually instigated by fever, exposure to the sun, or a food like chocolate.

When you feel the tell-tale tingle, get Abreva. It's the only nonprescription product with docosanol, which works by modifying the skin cell membranes, creating a barrier that prevents the cold sore virus from penetrating healthy cells.

Canker sores are quite different from cold sores, though people frequently use the terms inter-changeably. Cankers aren't contagious. They're ulcers that typically occur in the soft tissues inside the mouth and can be quite painful. They take about 13 days to disappear. To kill the pain, use Colgate Orabase Soothe-N-Seal, a gel that contains 2-octyl-cyanoacrylate, which seals off the nerve endings that trigger the pain.

COUGH
➡ Fight back with **dextromethorphan and guaifenesin.**

You'll want to keep these two kinds of cough medicines on hand because they treat two different types of coughs.

For tickles that produce dry, hacking coughs, use the cough suppressant dextro-methorphan hydrobro-mide. Fifteen milligrams (mg) of dextromethorphan every 4 hours should work wonders on an annoying cough. Look for Robitussin CoughGels Long-Acting.

For coughs with phlegm, use the expectorant guaifenesin. It helps thin and loosen the mucus in your

Q. How bad is it to take medication that's past its expiration date?

It's not as bad as it sounds. Most medications, when stored under ideal conditions (i.e., climates without swings in temperature or humidity), retain their potency for at least 1 year after their expiration dates, according to a recent study by the Center for Drug Evaluation and Research. But few people store their medications in ideal conditions. The bathroom medicine cabinet, for example, exposes them to extreme humidity every time you take a shower. Kitchen cabinets, for their part, can bake the potency right out of the meds if they're located too close to the stove. The best place to store your drugs: a kitchen cabinet as far away from the stove, and children, as possible. A warning: If you have old tetracycline lying around, throw it out now. Past its expiration date, it degrades into a form that can cause kidney damage.

— **EVELYN HERMES-DESANTIS, PHARMD,** *a clinical associate professor at the Ernest Mario School of Pharmacy at Rutgers, The State University of New Jersey*

lungs, making it easier to hack up. Drinking a lot of water between doses will help the medicine work best. Look for Maximum Strength Mucinex, an extended release bi-layer tablet containing 1,200 mg of guaifenesin, which lasts 12 hours. Once the phlegm is gone, you shouldn't feel the need to cough.

Avoid products containing both dextromethorphan and guaifenesin. While a dual attack seems appealing, the suppressant drug will actually hamper your body's attempt to cough up phlegm. Use a medicine containing both ingredients only if your cough is keeping you awake.

CUTS AND SCRAPES

➡ Fight back with **polymyxin and bacitracin.**

These are topical antibiotics available in ointment form, and they are all the germ-fighters you'll need for anything but gaping wounds. Avoid the triple-antibiotic ointments; the extra drug neomycin can sometimes cause allergic reactions. Look for Polysporin ointment or a generic. Apply a fresh coat up to three times daily.

DIARRHEA
➡ Fight back with **loperamide HCL.**

Getting "the runs" is often your body's way of flushing bad stuff out of your body in a hurry. Sometimes the best thing to do is just stay close to a toilet and wait it out. But if you must put the brakes on your bowels, loperamide will reduce the frequency of bowel contractions so your body can absorb the excess water that's flushing your intestines clean.

Look for Imodium A-D or generic loperamide. Bismuth subsalicylate, the active ingredient in Pepto-Bismol, is not as strong as loperamide, but it's a tried-and-true antidiarrheal.

FEVER
➡ Fight back with **acetaminophen.**

When a fever spikes, 500 mg of Tylenol Extra Strength or a generic will cool your temperature a few degrees.

Acetaminophen is easier on the stomach than aspirin, ibuprofen, and naproxen, and it's more accommodating to other cold and flu medications.

HEADACHE
➡ Fight back with **aspirin, acetaminophen, ibuprofen.**

All of the above will provide relief. Experiment with each to see which works best for you.

If the headache is really bad or you suffer from occasional migraines, try a pain reliever that also contains caffeine (like some variations of Excedrin, Advil, and Motrin), or just wash it down with a cup of coffee or a big glass of iced tea. A study in the journal *Clinical Pharmacology and Therapeutics* demonstrated that 80 percent of headache sufferers who took ibuprofen and caffeine together reported significant pain relief, compared with 67 percent who took ibuprofen alone. Caffeine helps blood vessels to constrict, helping the headache subside; and it also helps the body absorb analgesics more quickly, bringing faster relief.

HEARTBURN
➡ Fight back with **Pepcid AC, Tagamet, Zantac, Prilosec OTC.**

If beef burritos, General Tso's chicken, or some other tasty food triggers occasional heartburn, think before you order.

Swallow an antacid like Pepcid AC, Tagamet, or Zantac before you eat, and enjoy your meal. They are known as histamine (H2) blockers and are used to prevent indigestion by reducing your stomach's production of acid.

Antacids like Tums or Rolaids merely neutralize stomach acid after your body has already made it. Get Pepcid Complete if you want to both prevent and neutralize acid.

If you suffer from heartburn two or three times a week, try Prilosec OTC. This is an over-the-counter version of omeprazole, a prescription medication used to treat ulcers and gastroesophageal reflux disease (GERD).

Omeprazole belongs to a class of drugs known as proton pump inhibitors (PPIs), and works by shutting down the acid-producing cells in your stomach. Prilosec can give you relief for up to 24 hours.

HEMORRHOIDS
➡ Fight back with **Preparation H Ointment.**

We get it—you don't care to think about swollen, painful veins around the rectum. But, as with the diarrhea entry opposite, you'll be glad you have remedies if you need them for these discomforts. The venerable remedy Preparation H, more than 50 years old, contains mineral oil, petrolatum, and shark liver oil to soften and protect skin and a topical vasoconstrictor that shrinks swollen tissues and relieves itching.

INSECT BITES
➡ Fight back with **hydrocortisone and benzocaine.**

For bee or wasp stings, first make sure the stinger is out of the wound before treating. Dab on a hydrocortisone cream like Cortaid to reduce the swelling; that'll relieve some of the pressure on the skin's itch receptors. Then apply an anesthetic spray containing 20 percent benzocaine, like Maximum Strength Lanacane or a generic, to ease the itch.

MOTION SICKNESS
➡ Fight back with **meclizine or dimenhydrinate.**

You either get it easily or you don't—or maybe it comes on unexpectedly while riding the Tilt-o-Whirl or in the middle of a party-boat fishing expedition for sea bass. Once your stomach starts flip-flopping, there's no stopping the heave-ho.

So plan ahead by taking one of the above drugs at least an hour before getting on a boat/plane/roller coaster. A single dose of Bonine, a chewable tablet that contains the antihistamine meclizine hydrochloride, is effective for up to 24 hours. It doesn't cause drowsiness as can another popular remedy Dramamine (dimenhydrinate), and a NASA study found that it worked even better than the prescription motion-sickness drug scopolamine. Look for Bonine or Dramamine Less-Drowsy Formula tablets.

A non-drug option is the FDA-approved ReliefBand. This wristband emits electrical signals that interfere with the nerves that cause nausea.

NASAL CONGESTION
➡ Fight back with **pseudoephedrine tablets and oxymetazoline or propylhexedrine nasal spray.**

Pseudoephedrine has a stimulating side effect, so take it in the morning, not at night. Before bed, blast your nasal passages with a spray containing oxymetazoline or propylhexedrine, which decongest nasal mucosa by constricting blood vessels in the tissue. Look for Sudafed 12 Hour and Afrin nasal spray, or generic equivalents.

POISON IVY OR OAK
➡ Fight back with **Tecnu Extreme Medicated Poison Ivy Scrub, Cortaid.**

Leaflets three, let it be. If it's too late, and you find yourself in a patch of poison ivy, oak, or sumac, wash with soap and water as soon as possible to get the toxin off your skin.

Even better, use a product like Tecnu

Q. What's the best sleeping pill to prevent waking up too early?

Before you pop a pill, evaluate your bedroom. Loud noises, large windows, and even your restless partner could be interrupting your dreams. Wearing an eye pad, hanging heavier drapes, or investing in a wider bed could make the difference. Anxiety could also keep you up. Jotting down your plans for the next day before you go to sleep can help soothe your mind. If you're still catching the sunrise, try Ambien CR, a prescription sleep aid with a core that dissolves slowly over 7 hours to cover you throughout the night.

— **STEVEN LAMM, MD,** *a professor of medicine at New York University Medical Center*

Extreme Medicated Poison Ivy Scrub or IvyCleanse Towelettes. Both have ingredients that bind to the plants' urushiol oil and get it off your skin quickly.

If you develop the rash, try hydrocortisone cream such as Cortaid to decrease the swelling that causes the itch. Just don't use it on large areas (bigger than the size of your palm) because too much could be absorbed into your bloodstream and actually irritate your skin. Large tracts of oozing rash can be soothed and dried using calamine lotion.

RED, ITCHY EYES
➡ Fight back with **tetrahydrozoline or naphazoline.**

Both of these drugs constrict the dilated blood vessels in your eyes, which are causing the redness and irritation. Put a single drop in each eye and wait. Your eye can't hold more than that amount of liquid, and you'll waste it if you follow the directions to add two or more drops. Keep your eyes shut for at least a minute to give the medicine time to absorb. Avoid using it longer than 3 days, or you'll risk irritating your eyes and making them even redder.

WARTS
➡ Fight back with **salicylic acid.**

This is the same ingredient that's found in aspirin. It's more concentrated in liquid or patch form for use on warts. The medication works by eating away at the raised skin of the wart. Look for DuoFilm Salicylic Acid Wart Remover, Compound W, and generic preparations containing the salicylic acid. It may take weeks or more than a month to get rid of the wart.

+VITAMINS & SUPPLEMENTS

IMAGINE YOUR DOCTOR WALKING INTO the treatment room and scribbling out prescriptions for drugs to treat high cholesterol, high blood pressure, and thyroid disease—without ever testing you for those conditions. Something akin to that happens all the time in the anything-goes world of vitamins and other dietary supplements, says Mark Moyad, MD, MPH, the Phil F. Jenkins Director of Preventive & Alternative Medicine at the University of Michigan Medical Center. Consumers see advertisements touting supplements that offer everything from memory improvement to muscular development to penile enlargement, and they start popping pills on blind faith that these claims are backed by sound science.

"I recently saw an infomercial plugging an expensive supplement for eye health," explains Dr. Moyad. "The ad cited a clinical trial that showed an improvement in vision. But what the ad didn't say is that the pill only helped individuals who suffered from macular degeneration, and when healthy people took it, the pill increased their risk for prostate and kidney disease."

The hype can cut both ways. Just as you should be suspicious of claims that dietary supplements will give you 20/20 vision, be skeptical of reports stating that they'll send you to your grave. A study published in the *Journal of the American Medical Association* made dramatic headlines a few years back, thanks to findings that high doses of antioxidants can increase your risk of early death. The study—actually a meta-analysis of 68 previous studies—found that the risk of early death increased by 7 percent with beta-carotene intake, 16 percent with vitamin A intake, and 4 percent with vitamin E intake. But it's important to put these findings into perspective. What the study authors didn't say is that the population studied included people who suffered all sorts of chronic ailments—from Lou Gehrig's disease to cancer—and in some of the studies, people were taking doses as high as 65 times the recommended daily value.

A WELL-ROUNDED MULTIVITAMIN WILL GIVE YOU MOST KEY NUTRIENTS THAT YOU MAY BE MISSING.

So the study doesn't prove that healthy people are at risk. It does suggest, as do other studies, that there's a threshold past which vitamin consumption can actually increase your risk for cancer and other diseases. Dr. Moyad says you can make sure you don't cross that threshold by being cautious and strategic about your supplement taking.

+ **Take less, not more.** If you remember only one thing about vitamins and antioxidants, make it this: A healthy person who eats a wide variety of good foods should take one low-dose multivitamin, such as Centrum, each day. Little else. This is true for the elite athlete and the desk jockey. Low doses of vitamins and minerals have been associated with the best results thus far in the most comprehensive clinical trials in the world. A well-rounded multivitamin will give you roughly the daily value (DV) of most key nutrients that you may be missing if you don't eat right. High doses of antioxidants in pill form can actually fuel disease by not allowing your body to build up its own resistance to free radical damage, essentially quashing your internal defenses.

+ **Get tested for deficiencies.** While one multivitamin a day is a good guideline, you can take a blood test to determine a more precise accounting of exactly how much of a nutrient you need.

One test available at almost every medical center in the United States is the vitamin D blood test (written as "25-OH vitamin D"). The recommended daily value for vitamin D is 400 IU, but recent research suggests the number should be higher, around 800 IU. You'll probably have to specify that you want this test, because it's not commonly prescribed by doctors. But the test isn't expensive, and it could point to a deficiency in you. Most experts agree that Americans don't get enough vitamin D, an important nutrient that has been associated with reduced risk of bone fractures; cancers of the colon, breast and prostate; and even multiple sclerosis.

+ **Check your plate.** You may be getting more than enough of a nutrient just by eating right, and don't need supplementation. A landmark 1996 study found that 200 mcg a day of selenium supplements could reduce the risk of prostate cancer. Today, however, selenium has been added to many foods, and there is at least 100 mcg now in most low-dose daily multivitamins. So, what was once a problem of deficiency could become a problem of excess, and excess amounts of selenium from that same 1996 study were found to potentially increase the risk of some cancers, especially skin cancer.

While keeping those points in mind, consider these supplements, which may be helpful for the 40+ body. Ask your doctor if they might benefit you.

B VITAMINS

➡ **WHY TAKE THEM:** While research is mixed, some studies suggest that B6, B12, and folate may lower your risk of heart disease and stroke, says David L. Katz, MD, MPH, director of the Yale University Prevention Research Center. B12 is one of those vitamins that become more difficult to absorb as you age because acid in your stomach diminishes and you need that acid to unlock B12 from the foods you eat. Big drinkers of alcohol may be deficient, too. Vitamin B12 is also crucial for brain function. In a British study, people

Q. Is flushing unused prescription drugs down the toilet harmful for the environment?

Yes. Tossing them in the sink or toilet is no longer advisable. Traces of prescription drugs are showing up in lakes, rivers, and drinking water, raising questions about harm to wildlife and people. Some communities are developing prescription drug "take back" programs. The government suggests throwing most old medications in the trash—mixed with undesirable material such as used coffee grounds, then sealed in a plastic bag. For more suggestions, visit whitehousedrugpolicy.gov/publications/pdf/prescrip_disposal.pdf, which includes a few best-to-flush exceptions to this rule.

— **RICHARD HARNESS** *is a consultant pharmacist and author of five books on evidence-based natural medicine*

with the lowest levels of B12 lost brain volume at a faster rate over a span of 5 years than those people with the highest levels.

➡ **HOW MUCH TO TAKE:** 400 mcg of folic acid, 1.5 mg of B6, and 2.4 mcg of B12 through a multivitamin.

CALCIUM

➡ **WHY TAKE IT:** You experience bone loss as you age. This mineral maintains strong bones and is vital to the normal functioning of muscles and nerves. One survey recently showed that 88 percent of women and 63 percent of men in the United States don't get enough calcium from food. If you're not consuming the equivalent of 3 cups of milk a day, you may need to supplement. Calcium may also protect you against colorectal cancer.

➡ **HOW MUCH TO TAKE:** 1,000 to 1,200 mg per day.

COENZYME Q10

⇒ **WHY TAKE IT:** This antioxidant has strong free-radical-quenching properties, which can slow aging and degenerative diseases. CoQ10 is a vitamin-like substance that's highly concentrated in heart muscle. Studies have shown a correlation between low blood levels of CoQ10 and congestive heart failure, but the American Heart Association has not recommended the nutritional supplement, citing the need for larger clinical trials.

Coenzyme Q10 supplements also effectively reduce muscle pain associated with taking statin medication for high cholesterol. A recent study at Stony Brook University in New York found that statin users who took 100 milligrams of CoQ10 a day for 30 days experienced a 40 percent drop in pain compared with those who did not. Exactly how statins cause pain is unknown, but many experts believe that the drugs halt the body's production of CoQ10 when they block cholesterol pathways in the body. As a result, there's not enough CoQ10 to help cells convert nutrients into energy, leading to decreased muscle function and pain.

⇒ **HOW MUCH TO TAKE:** Dosage ranges from 30 to 200 mg daily, but talk with your doctor before taking it. Because the vitamin is fat soluble, for optimal absorption it should be taken with a meal containing fat.

VITAMIN D

⇒ **WHY TAKE IT:** Vitamin D helps get calcium into bones. Up to 53 percent of Americans may not get enough from sources of D such as direct sunlight, fish, egg yolks, or fortified dairy, according to a report from the National Institutes of Health. As you age, your body loses some ability to manufacture vitamin D from sunlight. Also, the current guideline for 400 IU is considered far too low by most experts.

Vitamin D has wide-raging health benefits. More than 1,000 clinical studies show that it may ward off breast, colorectal, prostate, and esophageal cancers; heart disease (by reducing inflammation in your arteries); osteoarthritis; and certain autoimmune diseases. "No other vitamin offers protection against such a wide range of diseases," says Michael F. Holick, MD, PhD, a professor at the Boston University School of Medicine.

➡ **HOW MUCH TO TAKE:** 1,000 IU from a supplement and multivitamin per day.

FISH OIL, THE OMEGA-3 FATTY ACIDS (EPA AND DHA)

➡ **WHY TAKE IT:** Fish oil has anti-inflammatory and mood-elevating effects. It's the only dietary supplement consistently shown in clinical trials to prevent heart-attack death by stabilizing the heart's electrical system.

Found in oily fish like salmon, tuna, and mackerel, omega-3 acids are known to lower blood pressure and triglycerides and slow the buildup of arterial plaque. It's been shown also that they relieve depression as effectively as anti-depressant medications and reduce the risk of cognitive decline.

➡ **HOW MUCH TO TAKE:** 1,000 mg of EPA and DHA combined.

MAGNESIUM

➡ **WHY TAKE IT:** A study in the *Journal of the American College of Nutrition* found that low levels of magnesium may increase your blood levels of C-reactive protein, a key marker of heart disease. Nutrition surveys reveal that men get only about 80 percent of the recommended 400 mg of magnesium a day. And the Harvard Women's Health Study found that women with adequate magnesium levels are significantly less likely to develop type 2 diabetes. The 40+ body is less able to absorb the mineral from food, and common medications like diuretics and antibiotics can further limit absorption, so you may benefit from a booster.

➡ **HOW MUCH TO TAKE:** 250 mg should do, as you already get some from the food you eat.

PLANT STEROLS OR STANOLS

➡ **WHY TAKE IT:** These natural compounds reduce LDL (bad) cholesterol by as much as 20 percent, which is comparable to the effects of statin drugs. Cholesterol also accelerates the formation of the plaques that are associated with dementia. You can get plant sterols in a margarine-like spread such as Benecol or in capsule form.

➡ **HOW MUCH TO TAKE:** 2 to 3 mg a day, eaten with meals.

RESVERATROL

➡ **WHY TAKE IT:** This flavonoid found in red grape skins, grape juice, and red wine has powerful health benefits, including slowing the growth of cancer, reducing inflammation, and fighting age-related mental decline. In experiments at Harvard Medical School, researcher David Sinclair, PhD, discovered that a specific enzyme known as a sirtuin could be activated with resveratrol. That's significant because, when activated, sirtuins have been shown to invigorate mitochondria, the powerhouses of our cells. In later studies Sinclair and other researchers found that giving lab mice large doses of resveratrol made them healthier and energetic, and boosted muscle strength and endurance. Most surprisingly, in some cases, it extended their lives by up to 30 percent.

Don't reach for the merlot just yet. You would have to drink dozens of bottles to get the equivalent dose. And some scientists argue that studies of mice don't guarantee that resveratrol will work in humans. However, the skeptics haven't deterred dozens of manufacturers from developing commercial resveratrol dietary supplements, typically made from concentrated red grape skins or the Japanese knotweed *Polygonum cuspidatum.*

➡ **HOW MUCH TO TAKE:** No study has determined an effective dose in humans; and remember that, unlike prescription drugs, nutraceuticals like resveratrol supplements do not need FDA approval. Until further clinical study sheds more light on the benefits of resveratrol extracts, choosing a reputable company's supplement is probably a safe bet. And, of course, you can get some reseveratrol and other beneficial flavonoids naturally by drinking two glasses of red wine a day or one or two 4- to 8-ounce glasses of red grape juice, and eating grapes, dark chocolate, and apples.

+INDEX

Underlined page references indicated boxed text